Becoming Reverend

Becoming Reverend

A DIARY

MATT WOODCOCK

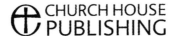
CHURCH HOUSE
PUBLISHING

Becoming Reverend: A Diary

Church House Publishing
Church House
Great Smith Street
London
SW1P 3AZ

ISBN: 978 1 78140 010 4

Published in 2016 by Church House Publishing

Matt Woodcock has asserted his right under the Copyright,
Designs and Patents Act, 1988, to be identified as the Author of this Work

The opinions expressed in this book are those
of the author and do not necessarily reflect the
official policy of the General Synod
or the Archbishops' Council of the Church of England.

The publisher acknowledges permission to reproduce 'Coat' by Vicki Feaver,
in The Book of Blood, Jonathan Cape, 2006.

British Library Cataloguing in Publication data

A catalogue record for this book is available
from the British Library

Printed and bound in Great Britain
by CPI Group (UK) Ltd, Croydon

For Anna, Esther and Heidi.
My best friends.

Prologue

Monday 27 April

So this is it. The next three days will decide whether I ever wear a dog collar for a living. About 30 of us are holed up in a large house somewhere in Ely. A panel of 'bishops' advisors' are tasked with discerning whether we are called to be priests. They've studied our forms. They've analysed our references. Now they'll monitor our every move for the next 72 hours. Our personal and spiritual lives will be explored in fine detail. We'll be questioned, poked and provoked in all manner of ways. It feels like Big Brother *without the swearing celebrities walking around in their underwear.*

Disaster struck from the moment I wandered in. I dashed straight to the toilet to unload some nerves. My fellow housemates were gathered just outside sipping coffee. I could hear them trying to act natural. This was a bad one. I yanked the flusher vigorously. Nothing. And again. No response. A wave of creeping horror swept over me. The shame of being turned down for holy orders because of a toilet malfunction was unthinkable.

Walking swiftly through the coffee drinkers to hide, I noticed a woman striding innocently to take my place in the stink zone. I should have warned her...

This wasn't the start I wanted. I'm determined to be myself here, but there is a limit. Our first task was to fill out a personal inventory. It posed questions like 'What do you think is the most important part of being a minister in the Church of England?' and 'What makes you

1

angry?' I want to be faithful to who I really am but it's so hard in this environment.

I led the charge to the pub tonight. Only one bloke came with me. He was handsome, relaxed and confident. He spoke humbly about his transforming work among the poor and marginalized on a sink estate. 'Tosspot,' I thought, shamefully. What am I doing here?

Tuesday 28 April

My priest pal Ben texted me some advice this morning. It said: 'Keep your head down, keep smiling and just don't get p****d!' I've been too loud today. I'm not exactly endearing myself to our assessors. Over lunch I happened to mention my former career. 'I hate journalists!' one of the advisors barked aggressively through a mouthful of quiche. I wasn't having that. 'You're wrong!' I spat back, showering his cardigan with piccalilli. We disagreed. Loudly. The other candidates on our table looked mortified. 'Keep your mouth shut and talk about gardening!' I could sense them thinking. In the end we agreed to differ. He later apologized for his outburst.

It has been a full-on day. I gave a presentation, chaired a discussion and wrote a mock pastoral letter to prove my sensitivity. In my first interview, I was quizzed about my background, personal life and sexual orientation. I think I overshared. Did he really need to know about me being kicked out of Cubs for biting Mark Low or my first snog with Gaynor Pickles in 1985? Probably not. The poor guy looked ready to blow his brains out.

A few more people came to the pub tonight. Masks are slipping. Guards are coming down.

Wednesday 29 April

Whether they recommend me for ordination or not, I have been utterly myself these three days. Warts, pimples, freckles and all. A lovely priest interviewed me this morning. He had that bookish Rowan Williams whiff about him. And a beard with things crawling in it. He said he'd noticed me clearing off to the pub, before whispering, mischievously: 'I was very jealous!' He asked all manner of questions about my faith and theology. I couldn't resist asking him about his priestly calling. It threw him. Tears filled his eyes as he shared. That was a bit awkward. But also quite beautiful. The guy was still crazy about God after years of tough ministry.

Whether I end up becoming a reverend or not I'll never forget this experience. I feel encouraged and affirmed about who I am, and what I'm called to do. If they do accept me for ordination, it will be me they're getting. Matt Woodcock. I'm sure that's who God wants. Not a slightly-watered-down, ever-so-nice Anglican version of him. He doesn't exist. I now await the Archbishop's verdict.

I got home and sank into Anna's embrace. She felt nice in my arms. 'Fancy an early night?' I whispered optimistically.

For St Paul it was the Road to Damascus, for me it was the A19 to Selby. Why God chose that day, that moment, that stretch of carriageway, I don't know. I wasn't feeling particularly spiritual or anything. I was on my way to cover a case at Selby Magistrates' Court for the *York Press*. I don't remember exactly what I was doing when everything went weird. Probably picking my nose, or flossing my teeth with a fingernail. I do that a lot when I'm driving. Suddenly my head began to swim and my stomach turned over. My Ford Fiesta became difficult to control. I pulled into a layby to try to compose myself. As strange as it sounds – and as hard as it is to convey in words – I felt an overwhelming sense that God had something urgent he wanted to tell me. Either that or someone had spiked my Pot Noodle.

This was new territory for me. I thought such encounters were reserved for enlightened monks in the wilderness. I got out of the car, sucked in some breaths and prayed. I expressed my confusion, my fear, but also my openness to what God might be trying to communicate. I instinctively knew it was something important – potentially life-changing. I prayed for calm until the shaking subsided. Then I remembered my copy deadline. Newsdesk had high hopes for this court story. I drove on to Selby …

I was converted to Christianity in my late teens. I woke up one morning determined to discover if God was real and if I could know him. Some of the people I admired most in the world were believers. They said they loved God. Not in a weird way. They were so 'normal'. That's what confused me. They liked York City and snogging and Regal Kingsize just like the rest of us. But they were different. They had something. Something deeper. A way about them. A different kind of attitude to life and people. A joy, a peace, a generosity, a surefootedness. It annoyed the hell out of me.

Eventually I decided that whatever they had, I wanted it. They said it was faith in God. In Jesus Christ. So I went on a quest to find him that day. I wrestled with deep questions, sought counsel from deep friends, prayed and waited for something to happen. Nothing did. I sat moodily on my bed that night, faithless and frustrated. In a fit of pique, I ranted that if God was real he had 'one more chance' to let me know he was there. I grabbed a Bible and randomly opened it. It spoke back to me. 'Ask and it will be given to you; seek and you will find; knock and the door will be opened to you' (Matthew 7.7).

Coincidence? Fortuitous? I don't know. But nothing has been the same since. The veil of unbelief was lifted there and then. It all made sense. I fell in love with God. His love fell on me. I ran downstairs to tell my sister. 'Amy, I've become a Christian!' I spluttered. She looked over at me with a withering glance only lads with older sisters would understand. 'I give it two weeks, Matt. Now b****r off, I'm watching *EastEnders*.' But Amy was wrong. It lasted. Lots of peaks. Lots of troughs. But it lasted.

Post Selby Magistrates' (case adjourned, as usual), I rushed to my vicar John's house to seek guidance. Before I could open my mouth, he smiled knowingly at me from his enormous study chair. 'Have you ever thought about working for the Church?' he asked. That was it. That's what God wanted to tell me. I've never been more sure of anything in my life. I knew God was calling me to leave journalism and work for him. What that looked like I didn't know or care. I was all in.

I sprinted home to tell my wife Anna. She was less sure. In fact all the colour drained from her face. We loved our jobs. We'd just got a big mortgage on a dream three-bedroomed semi within waving distance of her mum and dad. We were trying for kids. Our upwardly mobile life was humming along nicely. A massive pay cut and a crazy step into the unknown wasn't part of the plan. Picking awkwardly at our lasagne that night, Anna eventually said: 'If you're sure it's God telling you to do this then what else can we do? He's God. You'll have to do it. We'll make it work. Just be sure.'

My dad, a successful journalist himself, was furious. 'You're throwing your career away!' he raged. Mum was worried. Everyone else thought I'd lost the plot. My editor and colleagues cried with laughter – until they realized I was serious. Then they swore. 'You're doing *what*?!' was a common response. These reactions were understandable. I wasn't exactly the archetypal Christian. Newsroom life was intense, fast and thrilling. Bawdy too, at times. I thrived. My faith was always there but sometimes you might not have known it. Particularly on deadline. So the gear shift from news to pews wasn't ever going to be entirely smooth.

St Paul's, my local Anglican church, took me on as their community outreach worker. I looked up at the pained face of Jesus in the stained glass window on my first day wondering what to do. No one ever really told me. Stuff just happened. In my first week I helped a painter and decorator find God. Such was his apprehension about the church, our first meeting was on neutral ground – a bench in the local park. He told me he felt lost inside. If God existed, he wanted to be found. Could I help him? He wasn't alone. Spiritual seekers began to surface in the strangest of places looking for help. Sometimes even in church.

I also soon found myself combining my church work with a part-time role on the Archbishop of York's media team at Bishopthorpe Palace. Just months before, I'd interviewed Sentamu for the *York Press* about his enthronement as the UK's first black Archbishop. Sentamu inspired me to believe that the Church of England could find a dog collar to fit someone like me. I was encouraged to push the doors of ordained ministry – or 'test the calling' as important clergy in cashmere jumpers kept telling me. The doors kept swinging open. Meeting after meeting. Form after form. Test after test. Until I found myself in Ely for that crunch three-day selection panel.

I remember the phone call a few days later. 'You've been accepted for ordination training, Matt!' my church liaison trilled. 'The decision was emphatic – congratulations!' Anna sobbed when I told her. Then we both did. We were afraid.

I got a place at Cranmer Hall, a respected centre of theological training in the heart of St John's College, Durham. Anna decided to keep working in York. I would come home at weekends. The thought of leaving her wasn't easy. The timing wasn't great. Our efforts to have children had floundered after years of tests and two failed attempts of IVF treatment. Emotions were running high.

After my A19 encounter I sought someone to help me make spiritual sense of it all. Sister Cecilia lived and served at a local convent. She became my inspiration, my guide, my revealer of holy mysteries. She encouraged me to write stuff down. It would stop me doubting the truth of what was happening. I started a diary. At least an A4 page a day of musings, reflections and nonsense.

I get asked all the time how I actually became a priest. What was it like? What did I do? I suppose you'd ask it too if you knew me. This book – these diary extracts – are my attempt to answer those questions. I wanted to show – if you didn't know already – that faith in God is rooted in the good, the bad and the ugly of real life. Becoming a reverend was no different. For me, anyway. If nothing else, I hope this book proves that God doesn't call a particular type of person to work for him. He calls people like me. He might be calling someone like you.

So, I'll let the diary do the rest of the talking. This is how it happened. This is how I became a reverend …

Year One

Wednesday 23 September

It's my first day at vicar factory. According to the Church of England I am now an 'ordinand'. I'd driven to Durham with a heavy heart. A huge part of me wanted to turn back. I feel like I don't belong here. I can't see myself fitting in. Walking into the Cranmer Hall common room to meet the people I'll be learning how to be a vicar with seemed to confirm that. Anna gave me a despairing look. Everyone was engrossed in coffee and polite chatter. They seemed very much at peace. No one acknowledged us. No one. We stood like lemons.

I eventually swooped on a bloke called Phil. It turns out we'll be living together in the student digs. Nice guy, but I'd much rather eat my Frosties with Anna on a morning. After some awkward small talk we legged it to the Swan and Three Cygnets to escape. I shared my disbelief that God had called me here. It seems inconceivable that I'll last for two years. I reluctantly saw Anna off on the train at Durham station. It was like that scene from *Brief Encounter*. I held her close until the last moment. What have I done?

Thursday 24 September

Romantic, idealized dreams of living a monk-like existence in the community of my new shared house were shattered by 7.30 a.m. My housemate Dan dared mess with my morning routine. It irritated me beyond belief that he was in the shower when I wanted to be. What was he doing in there for half an hour? I seethed at the injustice of it all. I was forced to wash in the kitchen sink surrounded by chilli-stained pots. It's not quite what I had in mind for Christian community living. I stormed out to college with a face like thunder. The walk softened me. It's a glorious route through a wood and over a pretty bridge.

As part of community life at Cranmer it's compulsory to attend Morning Prayer in the chapel at 8.30 a.m. We filed in there with our shiny red *Common Worship: Daily Prayer* books. I'm going to struggle to connect with God in such a formal atmosphere of prayer. We laboriously recited line upon line of liturgy. It went on for ever. Passionate, poetic words of heartfelt praise were said in such a monotone, joyless way. 'As we rejoice in the gift of this new day, so may the light of your presence, O God, set our hearts on fire with love for you', we muttered bleakly. My usual way with God is so personal, warm and informal. Reciting Morning Prayer feels like I'm talking to a bank manager about mortgage variables. Deep breaths. It's only day one.

It's been a disorienting day. I feel like someone is going to tell me that this is all a terrible mistake and that I'm not actually meant to be here. In between listening to endless essential information about college life, timetables, modules and who's who, there was the small talk. Getting to know people is exhausting. I found a few like-minded people like Bill (who makes me sound posh), and Paul, an ex-army sergeant. I remained firmly within my shell, though. My appointed tutor, Stuart, seems to be something of a kindred spirit. He reassured me that God had called me to this place.

I'm now back in my bedroom hiding from my housemates, Phil, Dan and Clifford. I can't face any more small talk. My morning routine will now start 30 minutes earlier from tomorrow.

Friday 25 September

We went on a college-bonding trip to Barnard Castle today. I'd have preferred a game of ten-pin bowling. I sat next to a Nepalese-turned-Oxfordian called Sanjay on the coach. You need a degree in linguistics to say his surname let alone spell it. I think Shanmugaratnam is right. Interesting guy. He has a wonderfully warm face. Sanjay will soon be married to Menaka. Once it was deemed to be an appropriate match, the couple were introduced via Facebook and Skype. Sanjay says he has fallen in love with her. That's a relief. He told me that he's now looking forward to their first kiss.

After a service in a local Methodist church, we were left to explore the town. I went alone. There's only so much small talk I can take. I found a great chippy.

Saturday 26 September

Anna has come to visit, thank goodness. We ate a Tesco Meal Deal by the river. I bought her a Lottery ticket. She loves those little gestures. I used a combination of our past and present house numbers. It won £10. Result. We lounged in the sun by the water's edge like characters out of a Georges Seurat painting. The mood was ruined when a sheep dog jumped out at us from behind some shrubbery. I spilt my Quavers and Diet Lilt everywhere.

Tuesday 29 September

I got up with a new sense of optimism. I need to get involved and make an effort if I'm going to make it here. Even Clifford taking my usual shower slot failed to discourage me. There were no lectures after Morning Prayer so I went to the library to study. Bill was in there leafing through some church history books. We bonded. He worked in a factory for 30 years. His Yorkshire accent is broad and reassuring. We are kindred spirits. It's a relief that he feels as out of place as I do. Our bromance continued after college Communion. We led the charge to the Colpitts pub for the quiz with some of the lads. I've found a friend!

Thursday 1 October

Just when I was settling into college life, I'm now on my way to South Africa. It's a long-planned ten-day trip to represent York

Diocese which is twinned with three Cape Town dioceses. Our job is to strengthen the links. No pressure then. We represent all the different elements of diocesan life – bishop, priest, curate, reader, churchwarden, youth worker and more. I'm the token trainee Rev. It's not ideal to be whisked away from college so soon after starting. I'm secretly relieved, though. Anna helped me pack. I've left her love notes all over the house. In her shoes, under the remote control, inserted in the kitchen roll. She'll like that.

Our party of ten gathered at York Station. The archdeacon prayed for us by the flower stand. I'll be partnered up with a curate called Julian during our adventure. We hit it off, thank goodness. He looks about twelve.

Friday 2 October

Our group were greeted by a local senior Cape Town priest called Father Phillip at the airport. I caught a glimpse of the townships as we drove to Bishop Raphael's house for our first briefing. Cape Town is a city of extremes. Ramshackle homes are virtually next door to palatial mansions. I wasn't surprised that the bishop's house was at the more palatial end of the spectrum. Raphael was gregarious and welcoming. He treated us to a huge South African barbecue called a *braai*. The white wine was phenomenal. Julian and I are staying with Father Phillip and his family in a local township.

Sunday 4 October

Julian and I went to Father Phillip's church this morning. It was very eventful. They go big on the bells and smells, the bowing and the kneeling. Phillip's preparation was something to behold. He was trance-like. Woe to anyone who tried to speak to him. A sign on the church wall read: 'Talk to God before the service, talk to each other afterwards.' Six baptism families packed out the place. No one spoke.

Phillip had asked me to read the Gospel. No problem, I thought. Piece of cake. I was wrong. The choreography required just to read the Bible in this place was astonishing. Phillip's quick run through in the vestry beforehand left me utterly baffled. I decided that my only option was to execute the liturgical manoeuvres with the conviction of a man who knew exactly what he was doing. They weren't to know I was clueless. They soon would, though.

The time to read the Gospel came. I processed out behind Phillip. He held a Bible high above his head. I genuflected every so often to the weary amusement of the acolytes (candle-bearers) who flanked me. We suddenly stopped in the centre aisle. Phillip turned to face me. Maybe it was the cue to say my first line? So I raised my arms and shouted 'The Lord be with you!' It wasn't the cue, as it happened, but it made Phillip laugh. A cherubic acolyte with a devilish grin thrust a smoking thurible on a long chain into my hand. I was required to cense the Bible with three big swings. Three. Big. Swings. There were acolytes diving for cover, people crossing themselves furiously, Phillip flapping the Bible from side to side to try to get some of the scented smoke onto it. This was ritual – literally ritual – humiliation. The congregation's eyes were streaming from the smoke and the laughter. I think I did actually read something in the end.

Amid the comedy farce, there were some holy moments too. Phillip led the service like he meant every word. I loved the gentle way he baptized the babies. He blessed and kissed each one with the tenderness of a father. It struck me as we said farewell to people on the door that this church did not discriminate. For those two hours in God's house, we were one.

Phillip tormented me with 'The Lord be with you!' impressions all day. I preferred him in silent mode.

Monday 5 October

Our party has come to the diocese's vicar school in St Helena Bay. All the clergy from the area meet every few years for four days of teaching, encouragement, fellowship and wine. Lots of wine. On the drive down, Father Phillip launched into a rigorous assessment of my priestly potential. He said I was a 'terrible listener' and looked preoccupied when people were sharing with me. 'Sorry, Phillip, can you say that again – I was miles away?' I joked. He didn't laugh. Pastoral ministry would be a real struggle when I got ordained, he claimed. I admired his honesty (sort of).

We arrived at the St Helena Hotel to find some of our group were already tucking into the bar. Bishop Raphael got us to introduce ourselves to his clergy. After evening prayer we were treated to another *braai*. It took ages to cook so we stupidly filled up on liquids. The hotel garden became congested with slurring priests putting the world to rights.

I had a heart-to-heart with Father Stafford. He's a vicar in Namaqualand. Julian and I will be staying with him later this week. He's from a psychology background so he got all Sigmund Freud on me. Father Phillip overheard us. He waded in with more pot shots. 'You have an arroganshhh about you, Matt,' he slurred. (Tell me how you *really* feel, Father!) After too many Castle lagers on an empty stomach it all got a bit emotional. Tears were shed. They were mostly mine. I turned in about 2 a.m. I'm sharing a room with four large, hairy priests. There's no shower. It won't end well.

Tuesday 6 October

Today's guest speaker was a 90-year-old theologian called Canon John Suggit. He did three sessions based on his book *Mysterious Reality*. I was captivated by his views on God and the universe. Suggit critiqued Richard Dawkins's book *The God Delusion*, arguing that the Bible is all about the creation of the universe as an ongoing event. All life is one and 'seaweed is our distant cousin', he told us. He argued that reason and faith are mutually compatible. 'I believe in God but I don't understand him,' he said. He was a quote machine. I particularly liked these nuggets: 'Contemplate and then hand onto others the fruits of that contemplation'; 'Doubt bravely'; and 'Jesus is the vision of me as I have it in me to become.'

I enjoyed a riotous tea with a lively priest called Father Ossie tonight. A few seats along, Julian got into a heated discussion with Father Phillip. Phillip believes there are many ways to God other than through Christ. Believers in other faiths are just as spiritually valid as Christians, he said. I found Phillip's view rather surprising given that he crosses himself every time he stands up. Julian struggled with it. It was way out of his evangelical comfort zone. It seems that all our entrenched beliefs are being put through the wringer at St Helena.

I was cornered by an incessant talker at the bar after evening prayer. He had that uncanny knack of talking without breathing. I made a crafty manoeuvre and introduced him to Julian before legging it to the toilets. I came back to discover that all the joy had drained out of Julian's face. He gave me the death stare before escaping to bed. I was left up with the barman Leon, and three of the more alcoholically robust priests. We got the guitar out. They taught me Afrikaans Namaqualand songs until the early hours. I live for these moments of joy and wild abandon.

Thursday 8 October

I delivered a presentation to the priests this morning. In my talk, I basically warned them against complacency. I argued that our issues with church decline and secularization in the UK could be their issues in ten years' time. They gave me an encouraging applause.

One of the older priests took me to one side afterwards. He lamented that he was moved by my enthusiasm, but confessed to being spiritually dry. 'My fire has gone out,' he said. Bishop Martin and I laid hands on him and asked the Lord to restore his passion for the gospel. It was a special moment.

A wonderfully courageous lady spoke to conclude the session. She shared how her husband and younger daughter were killed in a road accident twelve years ago. He was teaching her to drive. She said that not a single person from the church went to visit. Her husband had been the vicar. Time had been a great healer and she clung on to every joy that came her way. We gave her a standing ovation.

Julian and I endured a seven-hour drive tonight to Springbok, Namaqualand, with Father Stafford. I love that the Anglican Church has a presence in this distant outpost. Our topics of conversation were weird and wonderful. Stafford posed the question of whether a tree is free. That took a few miles to get through. We arrived unscathed but tongue-weary. Julian is already fast asleep in the bed next to me. He isn't snoring, which is a lovely bonus.

Friday 9 October

Julian and I are getting used to each other's morning routines. He likes silence until he's fully awake. I missed Anna today. Dug out my wallet picture of her bikini-clad, standing in the sea in Portugal.

We visited the sights of Springbok. There weren't many. The closure of its once mighty copper mines has devastated it economically. The township had an air of bored desperation. So many of the people were sat in their shaded porches looking forlorn. It seemed devoid of any joy or hope.

Stafford invited four of his key 'church ladies' round tonight. Julian and I braced ourselves for stuffy conversation with pensioners in flowery dresses, drinking tea out of china cups. What we actually got were four Namaqualand versions of Beyoncé! They were wild, riotous women with filthy laughs, full-on faiths and full figures. Wow, could they dance! The gathering turned into a house party. They put on some pumping R&B music and showed us how to bump and grind African-style in the middle of the front room. Julian became a man possessed, busting out a series of thrilling dance moves. Their laughter and zest for life and God lingered long after they'd gone. My kind of people.

I stayed up for a nightcap with Stafford. He gave me this piece of advice: 'If you can reach the simplest person in your congregation you can reach everyone.' I'll remember that.

Sunday 11 October

It was like something from a Dickens novel this morning. I answered Stafford's back door to find four young, dishevelled boys. One of them looked at me with his big brown eyes, and said: 'Have you got any bread?' It knocked me for six. How desperate must you be to have to go begging door to door? I shouted to Stafford for help but he said he'd already given it all away. Rarely have I been so conscious of my own comfortable life. The boys walked on to the next house. I should have done more.

Tuesday 13 October

Julian's wife and kids were waiting for him as a surprise at the arrivals gate at Manchester Airport. It was a beautiful moment. Anna and I got reacquainted as soon as I got back to York. We literally ran upstairs.

I'm back in Durham now staring at Anna's picture. It was taken moments before I proposed on that rock in Holy Island. She's giving me an incredible smile. It's a look of hope and promise. Had she known then about my lack of sperm, would she have said yes so easily? I'll never know. Our childlessness is a pain that won't go away.

Friday 16 October

I read in Mark's Gospel this morning about the guys who lowered their paralysed buddy through the roof so Jesus could heal him. Jesus was struck by their faith. I prayed for more of it. Paul Bromley joined me for breakfast. He's had some life. He shared that he was once on patrol in Bosnia when the armoured truck they were in rolled down a cliff, killing three of his mates. It was a miracle he survived. Paul has a huge scar down his face. He found God as a result of the experience. I still feel paranoid that people don't really know how to take me at Cranmer. I'm not being myself.

We've got to attend New Testament Greek lessons for a minimum of five weeks. We can then decide if we wish to pursue it. I made my decision within two minutes. Learning this stuff is a baffling, impenetrable nightmare. To relieve my confused tedium, I tried to write down all the US States in alphabetical order. I managed five 'Ms' – Maine, Maryland, Michigan, Missouri, Montana.

This great Mandela quote inspired me tonight: 'One of the things I learnt when I was negotiating was that until I changed myself I could not change others.'

Saturday 17 October

I'm reading some of John Donne's poems. He was a saucy git before turning to God. I thought this was a beautiful way to sum up the base feelings of male lust: 'Licence my roving hands, and let them goe, Behind, before, above, between, below.' Anna presented me with some mini-gherkins as a special treat from the supermarket. The romance never stops in our house.

I texted my York mate Wellsy to find out how the Post Office FC boys were getting on in the league. He wants me back in the squad for next week's cup game against Tockwith. I'm pretty sure he just likes me being there for the laugh. My aim is to get into the St John's College Durham student team.

Monday 19 October

In our Greek lecture, Bill and I looked over at each other in quiet desperation. I lobbed bits of paper at him to keep our spirits up.

Wednesday 21 October

I made my footy debut for St John's College B team today. I scored our only goal from 20 yards out. It's wonderful to be back playing again. The St John's lads seem to view us trainee vicars with some bemusement. I'm doing my bit to change their perceptions. Being miles better than them at football won't do any harm. I'll enjoy getting to know these boys. One of them has already started calling me 'Rev'.

Thursday 22 October

Theological study has come alive for me this week. It felt great to hand my first essay in. I can't believe I'm being paid to study deep spiritual truths in the company of men like Bill and Paul. I had a God moment tonight while watching *Good Will Hunting*. I was suddenly struck by the awesomeness of Christ. It felt like, for a few seconds, I'd grasped the utterly shocking truth of his teachings. The parable of the Good Samaritan came to mind. It came alive in my heart. What a way to view human beings. What faith Christ has in us. What a manifesto for how to live our lives. Writing this, I still feel warm and funny inside. Jesus compels me to be a better human being. Not out of a sense of guilt but out of a desire to follow his example. If God doesn't exist then seeking to love others is surely the best way to live? It was a holy moment. Prayed that as long as I have breath, I will share his good news in a way that is relevant and real.

Wonderful Rowena from St Paul's randomly texted to remind me that it's my wedding anniversary next week. What an angel. She'd guessed right. I had forgotten. Again.

Wednesday 28 October

I get the sneaky feeling my housemate Dan doesn't like me very much. We had our first house bust up today. It had been coming. I'd innocently gone into his room to share a quote about Constantine. We got into a debate about the uneasy tension between the Church and state. Dan feels that Christians should never 'compromise' under any circumstances. I argued back that real life isn't as black and white as that. Sometimes the Church must pick its battles for the greater good. Dan is frustrated and angry right now. I challenged him that the answer wasn't to fume with anger in his bedroom about the state of the Church, but to get out there and change it. Perhaps my pep talk was too vociferous. Dan called me arrogant. He said I'd be 'useless' at church ministry. Ouch. It was good to see him so fired up, though. I hope there's no resentment. He's got a good heart. I must work on being less arrogant.

Thursday 29 October

Someone broke wind during Compline (Night Prayer) tonight. There was an audible vibration on the wooden bench I was sitting on. My money's on floppy-haired Owen. Or Gail. It was a lovely service, led by Andrew in his black, Matrix-style robes. Everyone went for port and cheese in the common room afterwards. I made my excuses and came home to watch *Die Hard* instead. Dan and I had more of a civilized discussion. He confessed to feeling a bit disillusioned.

Friday 30 October

There was high drama at the end of our afternoon seminar. The session leader said we'd finish by trying some 'body prayers'. A bit odd, I thought, warily. We were instructed to close our eyes and, when prompted, hold onto and pray for a different part of our body. As we got lower down – head, face, arms, stomach – I'm thinking, he won't, will he? He did. 'And now moving down to pray for our genitals.' No! The class did a collective intake of breath. My genitals remained unprayed for. I couldn't do it. I didn't dare look to see what others did. After praying for our feet we shuffled out in stunned silence. There was an understanding that we'd never speak of this again. Are they trying to get us all arrested when we get ordained?

I'm back in Anna's arms. We've been married five years today. She's still gorgeous. I bought her the new Peter Kay book, some pick 'n' mix and a bunch of tulips. She got me a lovely card with a poem inside called 'Coat', by Vicki Feaver. It says:

Sometimes I have wanted
to throw you off,
like a heavy coat.
Sometimes I have said,
you would not let me
breathe or move.

But now that I am free,
to choose light clothes
or none at all

I feel the cold
and all the time I think
how warm it used to be.

That's reassuring. And here's me thinking that she was sleeping with the milkman! After a heated debate we decided on a £5 Tesco Family Meal Deal for our anniversary tea. We should be better than that.

Saturday 31 October

I fell out with Anna this morning. Stupidly suggested that I was looking forward to putting my feet up in the holidays. Schoolboy error. She ranted on about how hard she worked, how little money we had, how she was making all the sacrifices to follow my calling. It descended into a full-on row in Durham's market place. Our childlessness reared its ugly head. It's always just below the surface, ready to strike. Anna said her colleagues couldn't believe I wouldn't agree to a sperm donor. I argued that I couldn't face bringing up a child that wasn't mine. Adoption would be preferable.

In the throes of an argument like this a storm erupts within me. We went to Nero's to calm down. Tears rolled down Anna's cheeks. Childlessness is like an open wound in our marriage. I can't face IVF again but seeing Anna this unhappy is unbearable. It's a worry for our future. We drove back to York in silence.

Monday 2 November

Edward Hopper's painting *Room in Brooklyn* spoke to me today. It depicts a plain woman looking forlornly out of a window. She looks hopeless and despairing. I imagine that she's a spectator in life, ruefully watching others living it. Her life is well ordered but utterly devoid of adventure and the mess that gets the pulse racing and the senses stirred. I suspect, though, like so many people in our society, she will remain at that window, watching but never daring to engage. Churches are full of women – and men – like this. What an awful irony. I feel called to encourage the Brooklyn window watchers to come out into the street.

Thursday 5 November

Joined my old colleagues at the Archbishop of York's offices for their morning Eucharist in the chapel. It's always a thrill to be in the presence of Archbishop Sentamu. He wore a very fetching Peruvian-looking woolly jumper over his purple shirt.

As usual, I got stuck in the hug/handshake vortex during the Peace. It always happens to me. There doesn't seem to be a definitive etiquette. Every time I instinctively go in for a hug, I'm met with a firm handshake. Limbs become entangled in an awkward wrestle as I try to get my arms over them and they fight to keep me at bay. From now on I've decided that if, generally, a polite nod is too formal for my fellow communicants and a hug and a cheek kiss is too tactile, then I'll go handshake with back pat. It's a fair compromise.

Friday 6 November

Our Cranmer year group has come away to a remote retreat house for the weekend. It's designed to help us bond and reflect on our calling. For the opening session we each had to lay an object on the altar that represented something about our future ministry. I brought my old press contacts book. For me, church ministry will be about investing in all kinds of people from all walks of life. My job will be to seek to love, encourage and draw them to Jesus Christ. I can learn all the best theology, but if I don't have a heart for the people it's all for nothing. We later broke into threes and had 15 minutes to tell each other our story. I overshared. No skeletons were left in the cupboard. My group lost the will to live.

There was some wonderful bonding in the bar tonight. It got intense and messy – spiritually, emotionally and alcoholically. We did impressions of each other and laughed at the insanity of what we were doing with our lives. After too many single malts, someone suggested a prayer time. We formed a circle on our knees while Jason prayed for us. Aidan burst out laughing. It spread through the group. Our sides ached. I'd like to think that God was laughing with us.

Saturday 7 November

Masks are coming off big time this weekend. It's refreshing to see people being themselves at last. I had a fairly riotous dinner with my table. We laughed at things we shouldn't and threw pieces of fruit into each other's mouths. After Compline, the female students decamped to a separate room to talk and pray through some of the particular challenges and joys of being a woman training for the priesthood. All the lads settled by the fire for wine and discussion. I've come out of myself in quite a dramatic way this weekend. Up until this point I've been unhappy and out of place. I've found my voice now, which worries me for different reasons.

I was left up with Sanjay, Jason, Aidan and Rob. We talked about demons, creation, evolution and what makes a genius. There was a real openness between us all. We've vowed to meet together at college once a week to talk and pray. The group will be called 'Morning Glory'. Happy days.

Monday 9 November

I felt called to pray for my York friends like Lee, Pete, Ben, Ian, Woz and Ollie today. We all found faith at the same time but I'm the one left still going for it. Surely they must still think about God? Reading about the adventures of a Catholic missionary called Vincent Donovan fills me with optimism for them. He worked with the Masai tribe in East Africa. After years of fruitless frustration he had an epiphany moment. He realized what his job really boiled down to. It sums up for me what being a reverend – or being a Christian to mates who aren't going for it with God any more – should all be about. Donovan writes:

This is what I and others like me are trying to do out there. Not to bring salvation and goodness and holiness and grace and

*God, which were there before we got there. But to bring these
people the only thing they did not have before we came – hope
– a hope embedded in the meaning of the life and death and
resurrection of Christ. It is a cleansing and humbling thought
to see your whole life and work reduced to being simply a
channel of hope, and yourself merely a herald of hope, for those
who do not have it.*

Amen to that.

We studied the results of our Myers Briggs personality test today.
To no one's surprise, I came out as an extreme extravert. In fact, I
got 59 out of 60 on the extravert scale. I am therefore categorized as
an 'ENFP'. It stands for Extraverted Intuitive Feeling Perceiving. We
are described as 'warmly enthusiastic, imaginative, life full of
possibilities, spontaneous and flexible'. I hate being labelled. Surely
we are far more complex than that?

Wednesday 11 November

We had our first Morning Glory prayer gathering this morning.
The five of us are so different. There was plenty of honesty and
laughter. Jason gets me particularly. I feel comforted by his wry,
knowing smiles.

It was my turn on the rota to give a potential Cranmer student
the college tour. I sensed the guy was only here as a token gesture.
His heart was clearly set on training in the South. It's a familiar
story. We can't seem to persuade enough future vicars that God
exists north of Watford.

Thursday 12 November

My struggles with Morning Prayer continue. We keep being told
how important it is to sustain our spiritual lives. Why am I not

feeling it? It seems to drain away all my spiritual juices. All I hear is a word-heavy drone. I wonder if we give God earache with all those words recited in that way. I crave something more joyful and uplifting. Like a hymn written after 1800.

Friday 13 November

Our pastoral ministry lecturer walked into the seminar with a freshly crafted side parting this morning. I stood up and said: 'On behalf of the whole class, I'd like to congratulate you on your new haircut!' Everyone cheered. He took it in good humour. Sort of.

Saturday 14 November

Back home to York for the weekend, I made the Post Office FC squad this afternoon. I didn't get off the subs bench. No change there then. The lads' changing room banter was something of a culture shock after being in the Cranmer bubble. I'd forgotten how terrible their language is and how filthy their jokes are. I've missed them. It was good for me. They are never less than themselves. I seem to learn more about God and human nature playing an away game against LNER Builders than I do in a dozen systematics lectures. As we got changed and rubbed on the Deep Heat, one of the lads told me that he'd stopped 'shagging around' because he'd fallen for someone. He reckons she might be the one. It's interesting that for all his weekly boasts of Saturday night sexual conquests, what he really craves is faithful love.

Sunday 15 November

On days like this I find it cruel that God has blessed us with a hugely enjoyable sex life that will probably never *produce* anything. It pains me that I can't fulfil Anna's longing for children. Driving back to Durham tonight I felt a deep pain inside. I curse my useless, useless sperm.

I'm increasingly aware that Sunday services at too many Anglican churches are just a bit rubbish. I long for more acts of worship that stir people. That speak into their everyday lives. Churches should be places to laugh, cry and rage. I don't find that enough when I'm in church. Worshipping at St Thomas's this morning was short on laughs, rage and tears. To me it was cold and tragically inoffensive. But then I chatted to an elderly lady behind me. She loves her church. It has brought her no end of comfort since her husband died. That shut me up.

Monday 16 November

I wasn't in a good place today. I'm frustrated. We are too often being exposed to an antiquated style and system of vicar schooling that will not halt the decline of the Church that I love. It's not Cranmer's fault *per se*. The staff are working their butts off. I feed off their intellect and infectious faith. But they have so many ecclesiastical and liturgical hoops to jump through to ensure we are churned out into the parishes with a distinctive type of Anglican cut to our jib. Many of us don't fit into that mould. We never will. Where's the risk and urgency and fresh inspiration flowing down from the top? If we don't start blowing away the dust and cobwebs of the way things have always been done, the Church of England will become the spiritual equivalent of Miss Havisham. We can't say we haven't been warned. This is what the official *Mission-Shaped Church* report says:

We live in a society, whether that be urban or rural, which is now basically second or even third generation pagan once again; and we cannot simply work on the premise that all we have to do to bring people to Christ is to ask them to remember their long-held, but dormant faith. Very many people have no residue of Christian faith at all; it's not just dormant, it's non-existent;

in so many instances we have to go back to basics, we are in a critical missionary situation.

It's pretty emphatic. We change or we die. The sooner I'm Archbishop of Canterbury the better.

Monday 23 November

I repented of my negativity this morning. It's not helpful to anyone. Prayed that I would make more of an effort to be positive and a blessing to my fellow ordinands and the Cranmer staff. Absence from Anna is making me much more aware of how much I love her. I fell into a deep sleep during Christian Tradition as we rattled through Monasticism, the Crusades and a bit of the Reformation. I fell unconscious at Constantine and woke to hear that significant things had happened in 1517.

Tuesday 24 November

I've received a rubbish mark in my New Testament essay. In his comments, my lecturer said I didn't know how to write sentences. Seven years of journalism and I still don't know how to write sentences. That's funny.

Wednesday 25 November

Jason announced at Morning Glory that Ruth is pregnant. I'd already guessed. We shared our hopes and dreams before praying for each other. Jason was in bits. He said his spiritual life had needed a group like this for years.

Dad came to see me in Durham this afternoon. We met in the Angel. He's the most interesting and interested man I know. The ideal pub companion. We talked about old York City players, our current favourite films (*Michael Clayton* and *Planes, Trains and Automobiles*), and Jesus. Dad gets so emotional at the very mention of his name. He has always got Jesus in the most natural, intimate way. The Prodigal Son story turns him into a teary wreck. He just can't seem to grasp that he could be loved or forgiven by him. One day. We ended up in the Colpitts. Dad was transfixed by the landlady's earthy honesty. Well, that's what he told me. She came out with a profound statement under his constant questioning: 'I wouldn't know what to say from your side of the bar.' We later met Joel Wood in the Shakespeare. More Jesus talk. More tears from Dad.

Thursday 26 November

At breakfast, I congratulated James on his use of the word 'ostentatious' in open conversation. Very impressive. I immersed myself in the life of St Benedict in the Cathedral library.

Friday 27 November

The experience of being at Cranmer means I'm constantly weighing up what I actually believe. My faith in God has always been so natural and child-like. Not any more. I don't seem to 'feel' Christ in the same way when I pray in the morning. I used to be so acutely aware of his presence. Being surrounded by such theological heavyweights is intimidating.

Anna cooked some delicious prawns tonight. We watched the *Gavin and Stacey* Christmas Specials again.

Sunday 6 December

Mum is 60. She still acts like a 20-year-old student at Freshers' Week. All the family crammed into a homely Italian place called Lo Spuntino to celebrate. It got very emotional. Of course it did. This is Mum after all. Sometimes I forget how insatiable her appetite for life actually is. Dylan Thomas could have been referring to her when he wrote: 'Do not go gentle into that good night.' Mum has never gone gently into anything. She's the queen of the ragers.

Amy and I paid tribute to Mum in a speech after the meal. I shared what I saw when I closed my eyes and thought of her. She has a Bible in one hand, a glass of Prosecco in the other; laughing grandkids hang off her legs; counselling clients are spilling their guts in her loft room. She's picking Grandma up from Acomb shops after a bath filled with candles sound-tracked by her soothing blue whale CD.

Amy's tribute was beautiful. We sang Happy Birthday while the waiter brought in a cake made by Aunty Lynne. I then stood on a chair, pointed to the door and announced: 'We've all had a whip round to get you a special present, Mum. Here they are for your pleasure and entertainment – The Chippendales!' Just for a split second she believed me.

Back at Durham, I watched *The Shawshank Redemption* for the seventeenth time. Andy Dufresne is right. We get busy living, or we get busy dying. Mum has taught me that.

Wednesday 9 December

For a supposed prayer group, we do an awful lot of talking at Morning Glory. The full rhythm of life is being played out among us. Rob plans to propose to Nat over Christmas. Sanjay is worried about his first kiss. Aidan and Claire are trying for a baby. Jason and Ruth had their first pregnancy scan. Anna and I remain childless. God has a lot on with us lot.

I disgraced myself playing for St John's 'B' team this afternoon. The longer the game went on, the worse we played and the hotter my head became. I was diving and screaming about like that PE teacher from *Kes*. With 20 minutes left to play, I was mercilessly cut down in a savage tackle. The young culprit – all acne and bravado – smirked at the thought that his studs might have hurt the old git. Every shred of Christianity seemed to drain out of me in that moment. We squared up to each other in a footballer's embrace. I grabbed him. He grabbed me. Our noses pressed together. Threats were made. The air turned blue. Only then did I remember that I'm actually training to be a vicar. I mumbled an apology as I let go of his throat. But by then it was too late for our team. My bad attitude had infected them all. Our captain ordered us not to shake hands with our victors at the end. So much for me setting an example! This is a disaster.

As a punishment, I went to Choral Evensong to support Jason. He was leading for the first time. The highlight was his announcement that 'We're now going to listen to a composition called the Vigilante'. He meant to say 'Vigilate'. At least it made the choir smile. And that doesn't happen very often.

Sanjay invited me and Rob for 'supper' tonight. I pointed out to him that supper is a pre-bedtime snack where I'm from. I also explained that 'dinner' is at lunchtime and 'tea' is the evening meal. His cannelloni was sensational. Once the wine flowed, I got the chance to gently raise my concerns about Sanjay's ballooning weight. I've been worried about him. He's a heart attack or a diabetes diagnosis waiting to happen. 'You're a good-looking man, Sanjay, but you could do with losing two stone,' I told him (gently). It turns out his weight has been an issue in the past. He used to weigh ten stone more than he does now and had to enlist the help of a personal trainer. I felt vindicated bringing it up.

Sanjay later dragged us off to Klutes, the local dodgy nightclub. I felt ancient busting moves on that student-packed dancefloor. I sensibly left at 11.30 p.m. with my self-respect just about intact.

Thursday 10 December

I'm still euphoric after leading Morning Prayer for the first time. I woke up at 5 a.m. panicking that I'd missed it. I settled in the front room to prepare. It's a tricky thing to choreograph. Praying has never been so complicated. Jesus must tear his hair out over the Church of England sometimes. I bet he thinks: 'All I want you to do is *talk* to me!'

It was a relief to get into the sanctuary of the chapel. Steve, the chapel warden, prayed for me after noticing my nerves. Everyone soon began to pile in. The Morning Glory lads squeezed me on the shoulder as they went past. My heart was pounding. I sucked in deep breaths. Then the chapel bell stopped, and the door creaked shut. That was my cue. I tried to be slow and measured, but do everything from the heart. It's the only way I know.

The feedback was encouraging. The warden said I was myself – but not too much. I like that. Jason said he was moved to tears. That's not unusual for him, to be fair. So, I've led my first bit of formal Anglican liturgy. I've learnt to not just read the words, but to try and feel them. And then try to live them. Here endeth the first lesson.

Wednesday 16 December

Sanjay texted me from Nepal to say he and Menaka had enjoyed their first snog. 'It was wonderful!' he wrote. Thank the Lord for that.

Dad and I visited our old friend Ronnie at his care home in Burnley today. He is always fascinating if frustrating company. Resistance to his constant verbal bombardment is futile. It's impossible to get a word in.

As usual, Ronnie loves to reminisce about his glory days in journalism and the time he came to stay with us in York when I was a kid. He took pleasure in reminding me that I refused to give up my bedroom for him because I was worried he'd die in my bed. It was out of my forced letter of apology that we became the most unlikely of pen pals. Not many ten-year-olds will have had one as glamorous as the *Daily Mail's* Rome correspondent.

After a few more wines, he chastised me for never talking to him about God. I'm still traumatized by the last time. Before leaving we exchanged Christmas gifts. He bought us a good bottle of whisky. We got him envelopes, stamps and pants.

Thursday 17 December

I met up with my Manchester buddies, Andy and Pete, in the city's Northern Quarter tonight. There was a lovely warm glow between the three of us. We laughed, teased and ranted. I got the tram back to Pete's place in Sale. His housemate Ernie (love that name) is a football nut. He has the great claim to fame of once playing for LA Galaxy's 'B' team. Pete cooked a stir fry. We raided the wine stash and debated Jesus, relationships and footy. Is there anything more important? And inevitably we got the guitars out and murdered versions of 'Half the World Away' and 'The Drugs Don't Work'. As dawn broke, I closed in a slurred prayer of thanks with Pete.

Saturday 19 December

I felt so happy today. Lazy mornings snuggled up in bed with Anna are such a privilege. The snow has made everything look beautiful. I walked to Mum's thanking God for the air in my lungs. I want him to know that I don't take being alive for granted. Having children may not happen for us but I'm still determined to suck the most out of life. Played with Phoebe while Mum and Amy baked cakes in the kitchen.

Sunday 20 December

My best friend has fired me after one lousy shift. It started well enough. I'd cycled to Lee's butcher's shop in the snow, after agreeing to help him out for the day. The Christmas period is ridiculously busy for him. My tasks were to vacuum pack huge gammons and brush egg yolk onto his pork pies (or 'multi-award winning pork pies' as he keeps reminding me). I discovered a real joy in doing such manual work. I lost myself in the task for hours.

Perhaps I should have concentrated. Somehow while stapling the labels on the gammons I perforated the vacuumed part. It rendered my work entirely useless. Lee went berserk. His face went red. He forced me to do them all over again. Then he gave me my marching orders. 'You're costing me money, Woody,' he said. 'Let's call it a day, shall we?' Fair point. I'll cross off butchery as another potential career option if I never make it as a Rev.

Thursday 24 December

The example of the former Archbishop of San Salvador Oscar Romero hit me afresh today. Not long before he was assassinated, while presiding at Communion, he told the people:

> … *nothing matters so much to me as human life. It is something so serious and so profound, more than the violation of any other human right, because it is the life of the sons of God, and because this blood only negates love, awakens new hate and makes peace and reconciliation impossible.*

What a tragic irony that his life was taken as he presided over one of the great memorials of love at the Communion table.

I had a very strange dream last night. I was at Cranmer as a member of Girls Aloud. I ran to tell Cheryl Cole that I was quitting the group and then called the *Sun* showbiz reporter to break the news. As I headed back to my dorm one of the students jokingly tried to strangle our principal.

I need to lay off the cheese.

Tuesday 29 December

Met my old friend Tom this morning for a brew. He reminded me that my faith and calling is not some academic exercise or pathway to a slightly fuller life. We get used by God to help transform people's lives. I had a lovely hour with him. He unburdened himself. As we got up to leave he grabbed my arm. 'I've got something important to tell you, Matt,' he said (rather dramatically for Tom, it must be said).

Instinctively, cynical old me thought, 'Oh crap, he's back on the bottle.' I was wrong. He said that Christmas at home with his parents had been a huge struggle. Stuff from the past resurfaced. During a moment of particular tension, Tom said he turned to his mum in the kitchen and told her, almost absent-mindedly: 'I could drink that bottle of scotch right now.' Staring at me with real fervour in his eyes, he said: 'The thing is, Matt, I realized in that moment that I don't need to drink any more because I'm now stood on a rock. I have my faith. Thank you so much.'

My heart soared. This man has been transformed by Jesus Christ. It has taken a few years and his daily battle goes on. But from where he was and the state he was in, it's a remarkable turnaround. I remember his darkest days only too well. On his way out, Tom embraced me. That did shock me. He's not the hugging type.

Year Two

Friday 1 January

A new adventure begins. So many lessons to learn from last year. So much I'm striving for inwardly and outwardly. Anna suggested that at the end of every day I should recall a moment of joy. She reckons that no matter how dark, depressing or annoying the day, there will always have been something to lift my mood, lighten my step and quicken my heart. I like it. I'll try it. Today I was struck by the realization that Anna absolutely loved me. She desired nothing more than to spend all day with me. That felt nice. That brought joy. It's a good start.

My New Year's resolutions remain the same as always – get closer to God and closer to Anna. I could also try to be less up and down emotionally. After 34 years of failure it's a long shot. Anna and I had a classic lazy day. We tucked into seven episodes of *Lost*. It's TV heroin.

Monday 4 January

I entered a prison for the first time today. I went to HMP Hull to visit Darren. I'm so frustrated he's back in here after all the time I and others invested in him during my years working at St Paul's. I tried not to show it. It was an affecting, important experience.

At the prison, after a thorough body search, we were herded into a waiting room. The atmosphere was thick with desperation. World-weary young mums fed their kids Wotsits to keep them quiet. I bought Darren a Fanta and a Mars Bar. He was full of bravado at first but close to tears by the end of the visit. I remain full of hope for him. It was painful to watch the other prisoners clutch their children when the time was up. Darren is desperate to get out. He has a TV in his cell, access to sport and a gym but he told me ruefully that all he wanted was to be outside and away from the sound of keys turning in locks. He held me tightly like a small child when I got up to leave. I prayed for God's peace and protection to be upon him. My hope remains.

It feels lovely to be off the beer and wine for a while. Sustained periods of abstinence are really healthy for me. My commitment to a Christian life of 'prayer and parties' is as strong as ever, though. I just need to get better at the prayer.

Thursday 7 January

I was relieved to get home from the cinema alive with Lee tonight. It was one of our crazy, magical nights. We inhabit our own little world. When we're not falling out, being with Lee is a gift. I don't know anyone funnier. It's like stepping back into those whimsical early teenage years. Cynicism, mundanity and maturity are yet to take root in our friendship. As we left Vue the snow was coming down in huge clumps. We'd seen *Avatar* in 3D. Lee said it was the greatest cinematic experience of his life (in the voice of an American sportscaster). His hyperbole was justified for once. Driving home, conditions worsened. I completely lost it on the ice at one point. Manoeuvring up the drive took six attempts. I'm delighted to still be alive.

Friday 8 January

There are times when I long to be a dad. Tonight's sledging adventure with the Mayhew family was one of them. I'd arranged to meet the Mayhew boys and Matty and Lee at the grass slopes outside Poppy Road School. I watched the way Ian looked at his sons as they screamed for joy down the hill. It's too awful to imagine that I'll never have a child to watch like that. We need a miracle.

Saturday 9 January

I'm mentally preparing for my return to Cranmer. It concerns me that Anna and I haven't made love for a while. It doesn't help that she goes to bed earlier than me these days. The lure of *Match of the Day* was stronger tonight. That's a worry. We'll see what happens tomorrow. The lure of *Songs of Praise* is not so strong.

Tuesday 12 January

I've been bouncing around with joy in my heart today. I'm excited to be back at college. Paul Bromley is teaching me the Book of Common Prayer's singing parts. I'm leading it on Thursday morning. The Powers that Be have decided we need to go even further back in time to prepare for the priesthood. I'll get a nose bleed if we actually lead anything written this century. We went up and down the relevant scales in Paul's room. I sound dreadfully out of key. I love the fact that Paul has an Iron Maiden poster over his bed.

Wednesday 13 January

Morning Glory has got very real. We are opening ourselves up in deep ways. We're tentatively learning to be vulnerable with each other. Jason is struggling. He feels down. He doubts his calling to ordination right now. He wept as I prayed that God would restore him. It turns out that he has a bit of a history of withdrawing into himself. Sanjay told us about his first kiss with Menaka. Rob shared how he proposed to Nat. Aidan said that Claire had gone into hospital because just doing OK is not good enough when you have cystic fibrosis. They are desperate for children but it could actually kill her if she gets pregnant. We all find it reassuring that God is in all of this. In the darkness and the light.

Thursday 14 January

I got up at 5.30 a.m. to practise my Book of Common Prayer singing parts. Surely there's nothing 'common' about these prayers any more? The old-English-style liturgy might be beautiful, atmospheric and even spiritually profound, but it is as common and accessible to my mates in the Fox as Swahili. And yet, secretly, I love the challenge of leading it.

I arrived at the chapel early to focus. Paul Bromley lent me his tuning fork to make sure I hit that crucial first note in the right key. The only place hard enough to make it vibrate when you're up leading is the side of your head. That felt a bit weird. 'O Lord, open thou our lips,' I sang. The rest of it is a blur. The warden's feedback was encouraging. They said that when I pray it feels like the congregation is invited into a special moment between myself and God. I don't know about that, but singing the Book of Common Prayer is another thing to add to my list of things I hope and pray that I never have to do again.

Tuesday 19 January

I skipped Morning Prayer and settled down with an episode of *The West Wing*, my Bible and some toast. Bliss. We looked at evangelism in our mission lecture. I was surprised and disappointed that so many of my fellow ordinands seemed uncomfortable with the whole idea of it. A room full of future vicars are struggling with the thought of sharing with others the faith – the good news – that they've committed their lives to. It's a worry.

I got into a discussion about homosexuality with Neil over lunch. I was delicate and sensitive. For once. It was helpful to try to understand his perspective. Defining which theological wing of the Church you belong to is important to people here. I don't know what I am any more. It depends what mood I'm in. Conservative, liberal, evangelical – they all frustrate me for different reasons. I'm whatever Jesus is.

On the way to lectures I turned the lights off on Jason enthroned on the college toilets. It was schoolboy behaviour. It shouldn't have made me laugh so much. Jason wasn't happy.

Wednesday 20 January

At Morning Glory, Rob said he felt called to pray for me and Anna over our childlessness. All the guys laid hands on me. Thankfully not directly on the affected area.

Thursday 21 January

Joel Wood led Morning Prayer with such passion and feeling. His words had power. His eyes blazed. Joel wouldn't look out of place living in the desert dressed in animal skins and eating locusts. He has got such a presence of God about him. During his prayers, he kept using the word 'fragility'. It spoke to me. I understood.

Monday 25 January

No one seemed particularly happy at college today. Jason is in a bad way. I'm worried he might drop out. I've been reading some more of Donne's poems. They swing from the salacious to the sacred. One of his holy sonnets brilliantly articulates the work of the Trinity in his life. I identified with every word of it. Amazing first line, too. It says:

> *Batter my heart, three person'd God; for, you*
> *As yet but knocke, breathe, shine, and seeke to mend;*
> *That I may rise, and stand, o'erthrow mee, and bend*
> *Your force, to breake, blowe, burn and make me new.*

Wednesday 27 January

Jason feels like he's being turned into an Anglican clone. His natural effervescence and freedom in worship is ebbing away. I encouraged him that we're not here to change how college works. We're here to learn what we can from the experience in order to be better at changing the world. Our own preferences will have to take a hit in the process. I'd love to work with Jason one day. He has it in him to cope with me. For a while, anyway. He cheered up in our seminar on diaconal (servant) ministry. We had to act out an embarrassing role-play in pairs. I hate role-play. The brief was to close our eyes and imagine washing our partner's feet. Some of the class got into it a bit too much. Tears of laughter ran down Jason's face as I knelt before him. His chest heaved. I forced myself to think some really unhappy thoughts to avoid losing it completely.

We marked Holocaust Memorial Day in discipleship group by reading some of Rowan Williams's reflections. They're so helpful in answering the question of where God was in the death camps. Many people want to know. Rowan says that God was in the innocent man who gives himself up to save his brothers in the camp. He was in the woman sharing her measly piece of bread with her bunkmate. He was in the son who forgives the Nazi guard who killed his father in the camps. Goodness and light could not be fully snuffed out even there.

I've finally enjoyed some success in a practical task at the house. The shower plughole had been blocked for a long time with moulting hair. Standing in there had become intolerable. I bought some pube-busting chemicals. It has worked! No more blockage. I feel such a sense of joy and fulfilment at my accomplishment.

Thursday 28 January

I plucked up the courage to talk to Anna about that which must not be mentioned in our house: the possibility of moving away from York. It wasn't well received. I explained that it could be the only way for me to secure a clergy job after Cranmer. Church jobs in York are hard to come by, I explained. Anna didn't want to hear it. The thought of being childless and away from all the people she loves is just too painful for her to contemplate right now. She ended the conversation quickly and frostily. She later texted: 'You promised that we wouldn't have to move away. I don't believe anything you say any more.' How do I fulfil my calling and make sure Anna is happy? There was a crushing sadness in her voice during our short discussion. After all she has been through with the fertility treatment, why am I adding to her pain?

I could quite easily return to the *Press* today. Life was easier back then. I had an exciting job, comfortable lifestyle, a wife who liked me, no Book of Common Prayer. I don't want to be a vicar. What am I thinking? The whole thing is a joke. I'm looking for some intervention here, God. You've gone quiet on me. You called me to walk this path so I'm asking for your help. Please make the IVF treatment work. Please bless us with children. Please make Anna see that moving away might be OK. I've got no moves left, Lord. Help me.

Friday 29 January

People keep telling me I'm a terrible listener. They may have a point. Our pastoral ministry seminar was dedicated to the listening art this morning. The irony wasn't lost on me that as our lecturer shared some of its basic fundamentals, I was texting. I didn't catch a word of it until Jason poked me in the ribs.

We explored the different ways that showed people weren't listening. Texting was one (sorry). Then there are the people who interrupt a conversation and proceed to tell you their own story. Other culprits are those who look elsewhere while you're speaking and those who just walk off on you mid-sentence. We could identify with the examples. We've all done it.

We broke into groups of three to try a listening exercise. One shared a personal story while the other listened. The third person evaluated how well they listened. Were they engaged? Interested? Sensitive? Sympathetic? Helpful? Scanning the room for inspiration, I noticed the listeners adopting a range of earnest faces. They tilted their heads to one side a lot. The only sound they made was that 'mmm … mmm' one that people use to prove their attentiveness.

I did my absolute best to listen to Jason talk about his dad for five minutes. Rob fed back that I fidgeted too much and butted in too often. I tried to explain that my journalist days had hard wired me to encourage the speaker to get to the point quicker. I'd learned the art of cutting in to avoid waffle. It enabled them to get to the heart of what they really needed to say. Or, if I'm honest, what I *wanted* them to say. Jason and Rob – in that lovely pastoral way that trainee vicars do – gently suggested that the listening aspect of my priestly ministry was not about foraging for stories but rather giving people space to bare their soul. They had a point. I tilted my head to one side, and said 'mmm … mmm', just so that they knew I was listening. I learn fast.

Saturday 30 January

Anna's time of the month is the worst time of the month. Always. It's a cruel, physical reminder that she isn't pregnant again. Understandably, her mood wasn't brilliant. Terrible, in fact. I got both barrels for simply waking up and saying 'good morning'. It's going to be a long weekend.

Tuesday 2 February

This quote by the theologian John Stott is one of the truest things I've read in a long time: 'In the morning the Christian rabbits pop out of their safe Christian homes, hold their breath at work, scurry home to their families and then off to their Bible studies, and finally end the day praying for all the unbelievers they safely avoided all day.' I'm convinced that God is doing stuff in people's lives all over the place. They just don't recognize him yet. I refuse to avoid, hide or cower. Wherever I end up, I will get out there and engage. Even with the dull and joyless ones.

Old Testament was a struggle – and not just to stay awake for once. We studied the baffling first section of Genesis 6. No one seems able to fully understand it. Who on earth are the 'sons of God' (verse 2)? Angels? Kings? When I get to heaven, God is going to have a busy few weeks answering all my questions.

I spoke to my sister tonight. Apparently my little nephew Joel still thinks I've come away to a special school which tries to turn naughty men good. He's not far off, bless him.

Wednesday 3 February

Jason and I are becoming real kindred spirits. We had far too much fun trying on clothes in Oxfam Boutique this morning. Jason bought a tailored jacket in keeping with his country gent look. I came away with some ill-fitting boots and a flowery, skinny-style shirt that looks ridiculous. I nearly bought a white fedora. What's happening to me?

I watched the final ever *West Wing*. My life will now have a Jed Bartlet-shaped hole in it.

Monday 8 February

I fought bravely to concentrate in Christian Tradition as we dissected the finer points of the German philosopher Emmanuel Kant. From what I can gather, he argues that God doesn't exist because we can't 'sense' him with any of our five senses. We later pondered the question: how do we *know* that Jesus exists?

Jason is in a bad way again. He reminded me of Dad on his down days. I'm so worried we might lose him from the community. He sent the lads a Facebook message telling us that he's doubting his calling to be a priest. We all have doubts but this sounds serious. Poor guy. I want to make everything better for him.

Tuesday 9 February

A day to forget. I said the wrong thing at the wrong time to the wrong people. It started in the pound shop. I asked a lady who I thought was the shop assistant for help in locating some items. 'I don't work here!' she snapped back, before storming off. Being mistaken for a pound shop worker clearly did not improve her day. Then there was our mission lecture.

We heard a great talk from the chief executive of Traidcraft. Fair trade is big business now. People love it – and not just the *Guardian* readers. I only have one issue with it: the tea bags. If there's a fair trade cuppa that doesn't leave an unpleasant aftertaste I've never had one. I've endured gallons of the stuff (and lorryloads of Rich Tea) at numerous church gatherings. This kind of selfish attitude, I know, provides scant relief to subsistence farmers on the poorer continents. And it's one thing to think it. There's just some things you need to keep to yourself at vicar school. Criticizing fair trade around here is the equivalent of singing 'Blue Moon' in the Stretford End.

By way of mitigation, I thought that to air the issue with one of the leading suppliers of fair trade would help the movement. I can't be the only one at college who has stuffed their Kenyan fair trade tea tin full of PG Tips? Anyway, never has a question in this hallowed arena of theological debate and reflection gone down so badly. You can question the Virgin Birth, the resurrection of Christ and even the existence of God himself. Raise the possibility that a fair trade product could be improved and you're in league with Beelzebub! I asked the guy: 'Please don't take this the wrong way, but why do your tea bags taste funny?' I wish I hadn't. Twenty death stares bore down on me, as the guy muttered a quick reply before moving on. I was only trying to help.

Thursday 11 February

It's increasingly dawning on me that I too often call a spade a spade – and then smash people over the head with it. I'm sure God is calling me to be gentler, less blunt. I felt terrible after the meeting to plan our mission weekend. I made the point way too vociferously that we were embarking on a faith-sharing weekend but not planning to share any faith. The rest of the group disagreed. They stressed that our role was to serve the local church and join in with what was already going on. It was a firm and frank discussion. My heart says that the sooner they all realize I'm right the better. My head says shut up and go with the flow. Deep breaths.

Friday 12 February

I woke up at 3 a.m. with a clear sense of what sort of reverend I'm called to be. It's one who is last in the bar and first up for prayers. Archbishop Sentamu is bang on when he says that churches should be places of prayer and parties.

I've finally finished my essay on the Oxford Movement. I won't get those hours back. It won't win any awards but I know what the markers want now. There's a definite system. A few juicy quotes of 'he said this' and 'she said that' followed by a not too controversial conclusion of 'and I think this' assures me of a mark in the mid-to-late 60s. Now I can devote more head and heart space to Anna and the IVF treatment.

Driving back to York, I thought about how I'd like to die. I think too much sometimes. I'd hate to just gently slip away after suffering a stroke or something. I want a dramatic death. A death with purpose. A front-page death. Trying to save a carriage full of train passengers would be good. I couldn't bear to pass away quietly in a hospice. It's not me. Anna had a prawn curry bubbling away when I got home. What a woman!

Sunday 14 February

Lee's mum has a new boyfriend – her first since his dad Ged died. He isn't handling it well. I know how he feels. Trying to act normally and politely when another bloke is canoodling your mum is difficult and awkward. But we've got to let them get on with their lives. Through gritted teeth, admittedly.

I enjoyed an exquisite afternoon with Anna. Her pea soup was a revelation. Quality home cooking is one of the great aphrodisiacs. By the way, I don't think God gets enough credit for inventing sex. It's in my top three of his greatest creations. Along with sea views and mustard.

I've cancelled all my meetings tomorrow. We need to prepare properly for this next course of IVF without distractions or pressures. Anna will be like a delicate flower in the coming days and weeks. I'm determined to protect her from the wind. We're still overwhelmed that our amazing supporter Martin has paid another £4,000 to enable us to do the treatment. It's not like he's close family or anything. He says he feels utterly called and committed to helping us bring a child into the world. His Christian generosity is off the scale. He must believe it will work this time. So should we.

Tuesday 16 February

I opened my eyes to a new day and our third go of IVF. The air was thick with a sense of unspoken dread. At breakfast, Anna and I descended into some mild bickering. We should have hugged or prayed instead. We were tense. Not much was said during the drive to the IVF clinic in Leeds. The route has become synonymous with the heartbreak of two past failures. Anna's hands shook as she filled out the consent forms. She's readying herself for a physical and emotional rollercoaster. I stayed head end as she was made to lie spread-eagled during the various checks and scans of her inner workings. We got the all clear to begin the treatment. Cursed my tightfistedness at only paying for a two-hour stay in the clinic's car park. Anna kept frantically looking at her watch when she should have been focusing on breathing deeply, staying calm and being positive. This will be a long, difficult journey. My sense of physical inadequacy as a man becomes heightened on IVF days. Why can't I produce more than about four lousy sperm?

We got home and Anna's dad came round. He waxed lyrical about what a gift it was to rock his baby grandchild to sleep. His timing for sharing that observation wasn't brilliant. Maybe in about ten months he'll be gushing about the grandchild we've produced. I held Anna in my arms when he'd gone. A lot was said without being said in that moment. It made everything feel better. I marked today's date in my Bible alongside this scripture from Luke 1.36–37: 'Even Elizabeth your relative is going to have a child in her old age, and she who was barren is in her sixth month. For nothing is impossible with God.' Nothing is impossible with God. Nothing. I flipping hope so.

Wednesday 17 February

I surprised my old colleague Mani today by turning up for the Ash Wednesday service at his church in Harrogate. It was a joy to see his large, beaming face again. Mani taught me so much about how to communicate. He opened my eyes to social justice issues, Oscar Romero and the joys of *The West Wing*.

I respect him for sticking it out here. It's a big, cold church with that air of respectable stuffiness we do so well in the Church of England. When I walked in, an old lady pointed at me and shouted: 'A young person!' She couldn't have sounded more surprised to see me there if I'd gone in dressed as a pink chicken. The congregation seemed to be dripping with old money. I guess that having a large Asian man with a Brummie accent as curate has been good for them.

In his sermon, Mani told a fascinating story about Archbishop Sentamu. When he was made Bishop of Birmingham he cancelled all meetings for 40 days so all his staff could pray and fast. What a legend. He's unafraid of making these bold decisions to shake people up and encourage them to get closer to God. The man is a prophet.

After the service I met Anna in the town. It was a bitterly cold, miserable day. We thought about going to Betty's Tea Rooms but the queue was massive. Decided on the cheaper Wetherspoons option but even this chain is posh in Harrogate.

Thursday 18 February

I think Grandma injects truth serum. She can't lie. If she sees it she says it. I've never met anyone so loyal, so brutally honest, so wonderfully inappropriate. She cuts through all social etiquette and hollow pleasantries. Put a few pounds on? She'll tell you. Having marriage problems? She'll ask. Large embarrassing spot on the end of your nose? She'll mention it. Anna and I had a thoroughly entertaining hour with her and Mum in Costa. Our childlessness was firmly on the agenda. Before heading off to her beloved M&S, Grandma said she'd been praying about our IVF treatment every night. 'The prayers don't seem to be working, though, Matt!' Brilliant. I love this woman.

Friday 19 February

I looked after baby Phoebe to help Amy out this morning. It was a window into what could be in store for us if my sperm get busy with Anna's eggs in the test tube. Phoebe broke me. I was assured she made not so much as a gurgle to annoy anyone. Then the screaming started. And it didn't stop. What a nerve-shredding, inhuman noise. I tried everything to silence her: toy-rattling, raspberry-blowing, peek-a-booing. Nothing worked. Seconds after Amy returned and attached Phoebe to her left breast, all was well again. I worry that there's not a paternal bone in my body. Not when they're crying, anyway.

Joel Wood is staying for the weekend. He's relieved to be away from the intensity of Cranmer life. I gave him a tour of some of my favourite York haunts. We did the Museum Gardens, art gallery and York Minster. We prayed for each other in one of the chapels. Inevitably I took him to the snug bar at the Blue Bell for a pint. We discussed what sort of reverends we might be and some of our inner struggles. Joel and I don't really do small talk. We plumbed more depths after meeting Dad in the York Arms. Joel opened up that he had once written two books on the missionary David Livingstone. He became so obsessed with the project that he eventually destroyed both manuscripts. They are lost for ever. I'm a better person when Joel is around. It's like having a pint of Black Sheep with Moses.

Saturday 20 February

I met up with the diocesan priest tasked with finding me a suitable first curacy post. We talked about what sort of church I was looking for. I told him that it would need to be somewhere fairly dead and broken so I could help breathe new life into it. Does that sound arrogant? I don't think I'm called to a thriving church. My passion is to see empty pews get filled. And then rip them out so we can put in comfy chairs. 'What about a church in Hull?' he asked. I said I was open to anywhere. I wonder if that's where the bishop has in mind? Hull will take some selling to Anna.

Tuesday 23 February

I've given up moaning for Lent. The only words allowed out of my mouth until Easter Sunday will be positive, uplifting and encouraging. All complaining, backbiting and mithering is banned. We had another meeting to plan our faith-sharing weekend. It was an important first test of my Lenten resolve. Our leader wants us to focus on serving the Church gently and practically. I want to start a revolution. My tongue is red raw from all the biting. I didn't moan, though.

Thursday 25 February

Jason has gone off sick with depression. Everyone is gutted for him. He's like our high-school quarterback at Cranmer. It had been coming, though. Sanjay paid him an awkward visit. Jason wasn't in the mood to see any of us. Fair enough. All we can do is pray. The college community seems to be in a strange period of flux at present. Gone is the early intensity and posturing. People seem much more dispersed and settled. Comfortable, even. My Lenten moan fast is going well. Seldom have I been so positive – and quiet.

Friday 26 February

Our Pastoral Ministry seminar was another belter today. We talked through various hypothetical scenarios we might face as priests. What would we do if a woman asks us if we think her husband is having an affair? What if we become attracted to someone during a pastoral encounter? What if they become amorous towards us? Being a reverend sounds like something from the letters page of an agony aunt.

Sunday 28 February

We've got another niece or nephew on the way. Rob and Sarah are expecting another baby. Anna wept when we got home. They weren't tears of unhappiness, but tears of frustration about our lack of news. Every pregnancy we hear about brings our childlessness into sharper focus. At least we now have hope. My heart aches for Anna.

We dragged ourselves to the service at St Thomas's. The guy on the pew next to me had a wonderful, rubbery face. I eavesdropped on some classic moans in the coffee time afterwards. One woman lamented that she'd been trapped on the pew next to two 'smelly men'. Another lady said that 'If that dribbling woman sits next to me one more time I'll scream!' The comments were made all the more ironic by the sermon we'd just heard about being more inclusive to the unchurched. Maybe the vicar should have added: 'Unless, of course, they dribble or smell.' It dawned on me that Jesus would make a beeline for the smelly dribblers every week. We too often do everything we can to avoid them.

Monday 1 March

A huge dawn moon hovered over me as I drove up the A59 back to Durham. Big moons stir big thoughts. They were fixed on Anna. She was restless again all night, twitching with nervous worry. It's the day she has to begin to snort the foul IVF drugs up her nose. I've ordered a mixed bunch from Interflora to be delivered to her office. They will cheer her up. Come on, Lord. Make it happen.

Tuesday 2 March

I know how it might have looked to anyone strolling past Bill's room at 11.30 p.m. tonight. Me, perched on the edge of his bed. Eyes closed, head bowed, palms open. Bill, stood over me, hands on my head, praying. In his underpants. It's difficult to imagine a profound spiritual encounter involving big Bill in his briefs – but that's what it was. I'd turned up at his room seeking prayer and counsel after a few drinks in the college bar. Shaking off his sleepy dishevelment, we were soon engrossed in deep conversation about the dark clouds hovering over college.

Bill believes we are under spiritual attack. Certainly there a few people off with stress-related problems. He told me that without our prayers he would have dropped out long before now. Bill is a lion-hearted, spiritual man, but the rigours and intensity of college life and the heaviness of his calling have really got to him lately. I'm hoping and praying that he makes it. We need him here. We wrapped up this holy moment with Bill pleading with God to bless Anna and me with children. His prayers stirred me to cling on to the hope I have in Christ. My friend is a great man of faith – even in his underpants.

Wednesday 3 March

I never know whether to shout, laugh or cry during our preparation for ordination seminars. They generate such drama, controversy and intrigue. Today's topic was the history of women's ordination in the Church of England. A lot of men behaved ridiculously and shamefully before it was finally allowed to happen.

After a run tonight, I stood in the crisp, cool air of twilight (sixth-form poetry alert!) and prayed. It felt like I was talking to the creator of the universe, my father and best friend all rolled into one. I can't really explain the theology of that moment but it was flipping awesome.

Friday 5 March

We're on our mission weekend. After a time of prayer in the local Methodist church, our team mingled with some teenagers at their Friday hangout. One of them told me that he didn't believe a word of the God stuff until he watched the film version of Dan Brown's thriller, *Angels and Demons*. It struck a chord with him. He now believes. I suspect Dan Brown would be fuming if he knew.

Saturday 6 March

Our mission team gathered at the local church hall to help set up for tonight's community meal. A wonderful old parishioner directed us like a grumpy military commander. We shifted chairs, fetched glasses and cups and laid tablecloths. I'm filming comments from our group about what they believe to be the essence of Christian mission. It will form part of our presentation. Rhys said this was mission – serving people. 'And I wish you'd put that camera away and start doing some, Matt,' he added. Fair comment.

Someone else chipped in that our mission was to pray for people. It was interesting that none of our group thought that talking to people about our faith – or at least asking people what they thought about it – was integral to mission. We love to call it the 'Good News' but many Christians seem increasingly reluctant or even embarrassed to share it. You could be left wondering if they really think it's that good after all.

Sunday 7 March

Our mission team took the service at Holy Cross Church today. It was freezing and they didn't have a loo. I was forced to relieve myself in a bush round the back. I found Rhys there peeing too. It wasn't the best worship preparation in the world. We had to wipe our hands with a dock leaf.

The vicar was thrilled with our input this weekend. He said we'd engaged with the 'people that I love'. His heart for them moved me.

Monday 8 March

Somehow I've ended up standing for the post of secretary of our Cranmer student executive committee. What was I thinking? I didn't want to do it with every fibre of my being. But then – annoyingly – something stirred in my spirit during afternoon worship. I felt convicted. It dawned on me that most of my fellow ordinands were contributing something to Cranmer. They were serving the community in some practical way. Being part of this place can't just mean pleasing myself. I've got to serve too. Being a Christian is so inconvenient at times! If elected, I'll be taking down a lot of minutes. I'll need to practise my shorthand.

We explored the Trinity in our Systematic Theology class today. I say 'we'. I was quiet, numbed by the discussions. My intellect doesn't stretch that far. Bill summed it up best afterwards: 'That were 'ard goin'!' Anna was really down on the phone tonight. She's been tearful all day because of the IVF medication. To my shame, I'm now nestled in bed feeling a sense of relief that I'm not at the mercy of her hormonal mood swings. I feel terrible for feeling very happy about that.

Tuesday 9 March

Mum swept into Cranmer for a visit today. She's a social tsunami. Take the most raucous, indiscreet, 'suck the marrow out of life' woman imaginable. Pour liberal amounts of wine down her neck and place her round a table with some joyful people. You're in for a good night. Mum met her match with Sanjay's fiancée, Dr Menaka. Talk about shooting from the hip. In the college bar, she regaled us with lively tales about training to be a doctor. Some of them made my eyes water. Sanjay is well loved up. He stared at his fiancée all misty-eyed, seemingly oblivious to her descriptions of where her hands have to go and what her eyes have to examine on a daily basis.

Friday 12 March

How to deal with difficult people was today's subject in pastoral ministry. The technical name for them is 'social tyrants', apparently. They have the ability to make church life and leadership an absolute misery. There's the aggressive types, the know-it-alls, the complainers and the gossips. Strangely enough, shouting at them really loudly to get on board or get lost wasn't one of the solutions. Shame. My hapless wingman, Paul Bromley, offered some useful insights. He unknowingly and repeatedly got our tutor's name wrong. She was too polite to mention it. I did the decent thing and held aloft a large note across the room, pointing out his mistake. His bald head went puce.

It's time to be bold and brave. I've asked the Cranmer community to come together and pray for our IVF situation in the chapel during Compline on Thursday. My tutor Stuart has agreed to anoint me with oil.

I received a letter from Tom this morning. He has taken my advice and started to smarten up a bit in the hope of finding a woman. He has come a long way from his drinking days. He wrote:

I am making a conscious effort to smarten up a bit, both physically and in clothes terms (not talking high fashion but just a bit less tatty). I'm fascinated by the thought of 'Woody' in clerical attire. Really look forward to having a proper chat about some serious theological issues.

He's finally ready for a relationship. He has been sober three years now. I'm so proud of him.

Sunday 14 March

Mother's Day. Anna was an emotional wreck. Full of hope. Full of dread. Will she ever get flowers and a card from her son or daughter?

Monday 15 March

Filling out self-assessment forms sucks all sense of joy and hope out of me. I know they're designed to be our shop window to future church employers. The problem is, I just can't imagine working for a conventional church or vicar. I'd do their head in.

We'd clash quickly and often. I don't feel called to fit neatly into the way church has always been done. I'm called to be a pioneering agent of change. I'm praying that God will find me the right kind of boss. A patient one who embraces change, hopefully.

Tuesday 16 March

My dawn jog with Sanjay was a fast stroll at best. His large bulk had squeezed into some eye-watering Lycra. Lord, have mercy. The views of Durham when we reached the top of the hill were far more pleasurable.

Aidan used all his artistic flair to create a brilliant representation of Christ's passion story in the cathedral tonight. He'd set different stations around the place where the different characters told their side of the story. They included Peter, a soldier, Pilate's wife and a priest. I hit the college bar afterwards. We ended up in the Wesley Study Centre for a late whisky with Bill, Joel and others.

Wednesday 17 March

You couldn't make this place up. Someone has accused Bill of hosting all-night drunken parties in the Wesley Study Centre. The cowardly complainant anonymously posted a letter under the door of his head tutor. The only thing Bill was drunk on last night was custard creams. We'd woken him up in his bedroom. Yes, some of us indulged in a few glasses of Glenmorangie but a night of wild, licentious debauchery it certainly wasn't. We were debating vague and mildly interesting theological concepts, for crying out loud! I long for a wild party but last night was anything but! I have my suspicions who wrote the letter.

Morning Glory is not the same since Jason went off sick. Sanjay is stressing about his wedding. The guest list stands at about 650. His father keeps inviting people. It's the Nepalese way.

Thursday 18 March

The college chapel felt thick with the presence of God tonight as my fellow ordinands encircled me to pray that God would bless us with children. Rarely have I experienced such a holy moment. Stuart anointed my head and hands with oil. A warm, comforting peace washed over me. I felt a renewed sense of hope that the IVF would work this time. It has helped me to believe again. Whatever happens, I won't forget their faithful, heartfelt prayers this night. They believe in the possibility of God blessing us with a miracle. What a wonderful community he has put around me.

Friday 19 March

I'm still buzzing after last night's prayers. I now have hope that some decent, usable sperm is beginning to stir. Joel Wood couldn't stop embracing me. He believes last night was significant because I'd been willing to show my vulnerability in front of everyone. I guess you can't get more open and intimate than asking a roomful of people to pray for your testicles.

We were treated to a brilliant lecture by a guy who co-ordinates deliverance ministry for his diocese. He is a real-life ghostbuster. In a wonderful Scottish burr, Raymond told us that his main areas of expertise were occultism, exorcism, ghosts and poltergeists. Ghosts were generally nice, he explained. They just want to 'go home'. He was so matter-of-fact about it all – like a mechanic describing how he fixes faulty brakes.

Raymond described the dangers of dabbling in occultist practices. He's seen people become consumed with an inner darkness. He is convinced that there's a constant spiritual battle going on, and prays for God's protection. His method of delivering a haunted house is to pray a blessing on it, splash around holy water on the walls and doorposts and command whatever is in there to leave in the name of Jesus. It nearly always works, he says. People claiming to be demon-possessed are treated with extreme caution. Apparently it's nearly always connected to a mental illness. Priests must get the express permission of the bishop in order to perform exorcisms. It's reassuring to know that there are ministers like him out there. I'm not looking forward to battling against evil supernatural forces when I get ordained. I still sleep with the landing light on when Anna goes away.

I've arrived in Arnside for the annual golfing safari with my York mates. It's such a relief to be with people who don't lie awake at night worrying about whether St Paul actually wrote the letter to the Ephesians.

Saturday 20 March

I barely thought about college or IVF all day as I just basked in the warm glow of male bonding. The weather was atrocious as we pulled up to Silverdale Golf Club. Before driving off we arranged our playing groups and ate sandwiches and chips washed down with a lager. At the first tee I gathered the lads into a circle for a time of silent prayer in memory of our precious friend Mark. It's nearly five years since his death. He was a special lad.

The most important thing about today's round was that I beat Lee. I relentlessly reminded him of the fact. Spending a weekend with these boys is soul surgery.

Wednesday 24 March

My attempts to stop moaning during Lent are faltering. It's a tough habit to break. Morning Glory teamed up with Bill's prayer group this morning. It was a bit awkward at first. We have different styles of praying and ways of sharing. We laid hands on Sanjay and Rob, asking for God's protection on their upcoming marriages. They'll need it! One of Bill's group is a wild-haired

African lady. She's one of the most eccentric people I've ever met. She berated us that not enough prayers were going up, shouting: 'Come on! We need to pray more! We need to soak this in prayer!'

In discipleship group, Rob Lee put on some chill-out music and handed out special soap to sculpt into any shape that might have spiritual significance to us. I always struggle to concentrate when prayer gets interactive. My mind wanders. I just about resisted the urge to carve out something childish. One of the women in our group really does my head in. I can tell the feeling is mutual. God calls me to love her – but do I have to like her as well? Surely Jesus can't have liked everyone?

Anna was a little spiky on the phone tonight. Her body is pumped so full of the injected IVF drugs that her hormones are going haywire. It's like being married to a member of the old East German shot putt team. Not long now.

Thursday 25 March

I was filmed and assessed on how I handle a difficult pastoral situation today. It didn't go well. A specially trained volunteer called Judith acts out a scenario that we respond to as if it's a one-to-one pastoral encounter at our future church. She was good. It felt like an audition for a daytime ITV melodrama. Within two minutes of the camera rolling, Judith had burst into tears and told me that her husband had a terrible drink problem. 'I'm so scared and lonely,' she said, 'Will you help me?'

I tried so hard to maintain eye contact and listen intently. I remembered to tilt my head to one side and everything. My solution to Judith's woes was that she needed to be in the company of some nice people from church. So far, so good. However, after being a virtual prisoner in her own home in the company of an abusive alcoholic, the last thing this woman needed was an invite to the pub. So what did I ask? 'Why don't you come to the next church social, Judith? We're meeting in the Red Lion. It's quiz night!' I'm an idiot.

Judith noticeably came out of character. She smirked in disbelief. Realizing my error, I looked into the video camera and splurged an apology. My pub invitation set Judith off on a quest to win a Bafta and a Golden Globe. She wailed and cried about her awful life. I offered words of compassion and sympathy but it was too late by then. I'd lost the room. I just wanted it to end.

Friday 26 March

I've survived another term. Everyone seems delighted to be getting away from college for a while. I'm growing to love the old place but it can be stifling, and claustrophobic at times. I need to breathe some different air for a while. I'm worried that poor old Bill won't come back. He was in bits this morning over his college work. Most of his time is spent looking up words he doesn't understand in the dictionary. It's not surprising, really. Bill left school at 15 and has barely picked up a book since. The irony is that he's one of the most spiritual people here. He'll make an incredible minister.

Goodbye Cranmer. Hello IVF.

Sunday 28 March

Anna's eggs will be collected on Tuesday. I'm dreading doing my bit in the sperm donation room. It's the place where dozens of men like me masturbate into a clear pot in the hope of producing strong-swimming sperm. I'm still scarred by the last time I was in there. Ripped remnants of porn mags were strewn across the table. Tensions are running high between Anna and me.

I'm reading a book about how to 'interpret' the Bible. It's a challenge to those who read it in a black-and-white way. The author argues that our holy book reveals God's truth but doesn't establish exactitudes. It's not a history or science book but one that's full of uncertainties and ambiguities – just like life. That makes sense.

I wrote a song today about a lad I saw in my reporting days throwing himself from a hotel bedroom. I've called it 'The Falling Man'. It's dreadful.

Monday 29 March

I'm on a primary school placement this week. It was a fascinating and enlightening day. The head summed it up: 'There's no better way to serve God than to serve children – even when they're sh***ing on your floor.' He'd had a stressful afternoon dealing with a troubled young girl. The school were struggling to control her, not to mention her adoptive parents. She had ended up in the head's office waiting to be picked up after a classroom meltdown. While in there, she defecated in the middle of his floor. I was struck by the loving, tender way it was handled. They're trying hard to prevent her from being permanently excluded. The heavy demands of teaching were evident in the harassed faces of the weary-looking staff. They arrive early and leave late and seem constantly up against it.

Tuesday 30 March

There's low sperm counts and there's low sperm counts. On the day I needed it most, my useless penis failed to deliver. It looks like we'll be doing the IVF treatment the hard way again. In theory, it should have been simple. The doctors would extract eggs from Anna. They would then take the best of the sperm I produced and fuse them both together in a Petri dish in the hope of creating our son or daughter. That was the plan, anyway. The specialist fertility section at Seacroft Hospital is so much nicer than its former home at Leeds General Infirmary. Nicer parking, nicer room, nicer everything.

The waiting room was as tense as ever. Anxious, hopeful couples fidgeted uneasily in their seats. There were a few noisy toddlers roaming around. They are a visible, cruel reminder of the thing we most desire in the world but we only have a 20 per cent chance of getting through this treatment. It was difficult not to resent their parents trying for more children when we haven't even got one. Childlessness does that to you.

In an effort to stay calm, I lost myself in the adventure of one of my favourite reads: *Modesty Blaise: A Taste for Death*. Its ingenious action set-pieces cancelled out the noise and tension. Delicata – 'the giant who is impervious to pain' – is still my favourite baddie of all time. Being transported into Modesty's world was a gift. I could have stayed there all day. Eventually our name was called and we were ushered into a small cubicle. A guy next to us chirped away loudly on his mobile about accountants and pension funds. He boasted that he could get his clients '£100,000 tax free'. I realized that this was his way of coping. I had Modesty, he had boastful conversations about tax breaks.

Then it all happened quite quickly. Anna was whisked away to have her eggs extracted. She came back 30 minutes later, groggy and mumbling about '18 eggs'. While she recovered I was summoned to give my sample. I had a bad feeling about it. There didn't seem to be much in the pot once I'd done the business. Later, the results revealed that there was nothing in it. Not one single, usable sperm. Unbelievable. And yet all was not lost. An impressive 17 eggs were extracted from Anna. The hospital will use some of my previously frozen sperm from two years ago. The quality may have been affected but at least they can use something. The odds aren't good. Anna came round quite quickly but looked very pale.

We got home and collapsed into bed. I later went for fish and chips and a DVD to cheer us up. The chippy lady put in a free tub of ice cream. I don't know why. It felt like a gift from God. A kind and wonderful gesture at the end of a horrible day. So, no sperm, but we still have hope.

Wednesday 31 March

I still don't know the technical, scientific terms for any of it, but somehow by putting together Anna's eggs with my frozen sperm in a test tube, five embryos have been created. It means we could still produce a child. The embryos will do what they do and then the best of them will be inserted into Anna on Good Friday. The significance of that day is not lost on us.

Thursday 1 April

Some of the staff at my placement school let their masks slip today. It's no wonder so many teachers are off sick with stress. In the face of Himalayan-sized workloads and endless targets and assessment, they have to spend their days projecting a sense of control, happiness and unflappability to their classes. It hasn't surprised me to discover that they're as broken as the rest of us. Too many clergy are the same with their congregations. It's all smiles and comfortable cardigans on the surface, but the plague of inner despair eats away on the inside. I must never be that way. One of the staff said he was still recovering from a nervous breakdown. Another teacher is bitter and lost after the collapse of her marriage. One of the younger staff is still getting over the trauma of working under a cruel and tyrannical head at her previous school. A kind and lovely member of the team apparently turns into a monster after too many drinks. I've warmed to them all this week.

I got a bit carried away playing football with some of the Year Six boys at lunchtime. That's an understatement. Every pass, shot and tackle meant a bit too much. It didn't end well. I stretched too far to tackle a small plump boy and my smooth-soled brogues slipped on some gravel. I went flying head first into the ground, scraping my cheek, ripping my trousers and smashing my elbow. It hurt. A lot. I may have let out a little profanity. The small plump boy was the first to laugh. The rest of the playground followed suit. I hobbled away trying to smile – throbbing, bleeding and humiliated.

I joined some of the staff for a pint after school. I needed one. Just when I thought I'd heard enough stories of brokenness and despair for one day, I got chatting to a bloke at the bar. Steve wasn't in a good way. He had been a successful bricklayer, married, with two kids and a nice house in a leafy suburb. One day he was walking along the street when he was jumped from behind by a gang. They smashed his head with a metal bar and beat him senseless. The police were baffled. It turned out to be a case of mistaken identity. Steve suffered a blood clot on the brain and fell into a coma. While he lay in hospital his business went down the pan. When he finally awoke his wife asked for a divorce. His friends deserted him. He spent many months failing to get legal help. Only now is Steve on the verge of receiving compensation. 'I know it's not healthy to be bitter,' he told me, 'but I've lost my faith in people for ever. I'll never trust anyone again.' I tried my best to be positive about his future, but Steve is still too angry to listen to words of hope. Where was his Good Samaritan?

Friday 2 April

My recurring nightmare became a reality while out running this morning. I noticed a young lad walking a very large dog – like a cross between a bull mastiff and that slavering one from *Turner and Hooch*. It broke free of the boy, and sprinted towards me with a mean look in its eye. I nearly filled my running shorts. Mercifully it turned back just moments before my leg became breakfast.

I could have done without it today. We had fears enough at our crunch IVF session in Leeds. Two embryos were inserted into Anna

– by one of the North's 'top fertility doctors' (so a nurse told us). She hitched her legs up and clutched tightly onto my hand. They went in successfully. We have hope. My job now is to keep Anna healthy and positive.

Tuesday 6 April

Aunty Lynne has got cancer. None of us can believe it. What is going on, Lord? Uncle Ally and Jo, Becky and Lorrie are beside themselves. Jo was still in shock when I called her. What could I say? The cancer is in Aunty Lynne's oesophagus. It's a tough area to operate on, apparently. It doesn't sound good. She needs more tests. I texted Becky: 'I'm praying for your mum, Beck. Love you all x'. She replied: 'Thanks, Matt. I'm just so upset and can't believe it's happening x'. They will need a lot of prayer and patience. I'm worried that I don't have enough faith that God will heal her. Uncle Ally must be so afraid. They are the closest couple I know.

Wednesday 7 April

I got up at 6.30 a.m. to pray for Aunty Lynne. I lit some candles and silently meditated over the situation. We will pull together as a family. I will be there for them. One of Uncle Ally's trademark phrases is 'I don't do bad news'. In the end, though, none of us are immune to it. I prayed that he will have the strength to endure it. We're staying positive.

Anna and I have come to London for a mini-break. Our adventure began in Hyde Park. I wanted to experience Speakers' Corner. There were no speakers to be found. Typical. Walking is the best way to really appreciate London. We took it steady as I was mindful that Anna could be carrying our child. Park Lane was a fascinating insight into how the other half live. The top-hat-wearing porter outside the Dorchester was typical of the grandness of the area. Until I noticed he was slyly chewing gum. We ate our sandwiches outside Buckingham Palace. I looked up at the windows, imagining the historic stuff that has gone on behind them.

As we 'debated' the directions to our hotel, a voice came out of nowhere. 'Is that you, Woody?' It was my old *Press* colleague Mike Carroll. You can't go anywhere. He now works in London for the Press Association. I still feel bad about the way I treated him when he was promoted to deputy news editor. Mike and I were too competitive. We battled many times to get that front-page splash. From a distance, it all seems rather sad now. I was childish and unhelpful towards him when he took the step up. Deep down I probably wish it had been me. Mike didn't seem to hold any grudges. He even confessed to now being a regular at church. You just never know.

After a quick snooze we met our old friend Dan Holmes in a bar near Covent Garden. He is dating a stick-thin society girl with a name that sounds made up – Clarissa Le Cash. She is personal assistant to a supermodel and her dad photographs rock legends. Now she's dating a York City fan. We got tickets for *Billy Elliot*. It wasn't a patch on *Les Mis*. The songs weren't strong enough. There was a terrible smell of turnips in the theatre.

Friday 9 April

Waiting for the IVF results is painful. We feel helpless. Anna is bouncing off the walls. We can't face anyone. My eyes are constantly drawn to Anna's stomach. I hope against hope that she's carrying our son or daughter.

I found consolation in watching the last-ever episode of *The Sopranos*. So, we'll never know Tony's fate. I have my theories about what happened to him in that restaurant. Anna and I later ventured out to place our bets on the Grand National. I've gone for the 100–1 long shot, Priest's Leap. It can't lose.

Saturday 10 April

Anna backed the Grand National winner. She pocketed £41 after Don't Push It romped home. It couldn't lift our blues. My pain is seeing Anna's pain. Her emotions are yo-yoing. It's hideous to see the torture in her eyes as we wait.

I tried to run off my melancholy in the heat of the day. I saw one of my old football buddies in the beer garden of his new pub, the Cross Keys. We high-fived each other as I ran past. Sometimes I love the familiarity of living in York.

It was a late finish at Beck and Matt's house party tonight. I niggled with Lee most of the night. I got deep and serious with his sister Nicola. She can't understand why God 'let' her dad die. I eventually wobbled home after busting out a pathetic Moonwalk in the kitchen to make the late revellers laugh. I've been doing stuff like that since primary school. Vicar school is so far failing to stop my craving to be the centre of attention. At least I've stopped shoving fat crayons up my nose and burping the *EastEnders* theme tune. That's progress.

Sunday 11 April

I heroically got up to fulfil a promise to hear Aidan preach at St Thomas's. The pews are particularly cold and hard at this church. Only an absolute sadist would invent such a wretched seating experience – and then put them in God's house. My poor bum took a real hammering.

With two baptisms on, it was a tough gig for Aidan. He wasn't expecting the church to be so full of people. They looked like they didn't want to be there. And that was just the parents and godparents. I wonder what God makes of these occasions? As church leaders, it's easy to become despondent and critical. Trying to communicate the love of God to a group of people who are willing you to shut up so they can move on to the Christening party can be soul-destroying. That's if they look up from their phones to listen. And yet. They are here. They came. In all their best clothes, new haircuts and spray tans. They came to church! What an opportunity. What a privilege.

We've got to work harder. The embarrassment, the lack of engagement, the desperation to be elsewhere, we can do something about that. God is too big. His message is too great to give up. He can penetrate the hardest of disinterested hearts. He uses us to get their attention. We must fight against the chaos of texting, chattering and disrespect, to create holy moments and opportunities. I'm going all in when I get ordained.

Aidan, bless him, was theologically sound in his preaching. He always is. But I didn't think this was the right time to talk in abstract ways about the power of the resurrection. He's a gifted communicator but if 70 per cent of the congregation have no idea what he's talking about then there's a problem.

Monday 12 April

There's only so long I can keep things hidden from God. I felt the benefit of some intense time with him this morning. He helps me open up the places of my heart that hurt the most. Like the IVF places. I stumbled across an old prayer book that helped me find words of honesty and repentance. I laid on the front room floor and poured it all out to him as intimately as if he was next to me. I told him all my fears and frustrations over IVF and Aunty Lynne. Then I just shut up for a while and rested in his presence. I came to a place of solitude and peace. Life takes on such a lighter, more hopeful hue when I spend proper time with God. It's crazy that I so often shut him out when things are painful and dark. Mornings like this remind me why I believe. I now feel ready to endure the IVF and keep believing for Aunty Lynne. God is real. He works.

There was a special impromptu gathering in Aunty Lynne's garden this afternoon with Becky and the kids, Jo and Uncle Ally. I held my aunty in a crushing bear hug. I wanted to squeeze my love and concern into her. I hope she knows how special she is to me. I'll never forget how, for a long time, in the maelstrom of our chaotic home life, she remained such a rock and a comforter to me and Amy. We were never easy kids but her house was always available for countless casseroles and weekend sleepovers. It was our haven. She looks gaunt but is being positive and strong. Uncle Ally had a haunted look. In a quiet moment with Becky she told me: 'Things like this aren't supposed to happen in our family.' At least no one is suppressing how they really feel. We're expressing ourselves with tears and laughter. That's our way.

Tuesday 13 April

Grumpy start to the day. The boiler man woke me up and then I had heated words with Anna because I couldn't find the sugar. I'm such a child. I've received an email back from the producers of an Oasis documentary. They're looking for fans to contribute something of what the band means to them. The quirkier and more interesting the better. They like the fact that I'm training to be a vicar. Told them that I'd used their music to highlight spiritual points during special services in the past. I may have exaggerated the extent of this, mind you. The possibility of meeting Noel Gallagher is clouding my judgement. Just recently I've been day-dreaming about helping him to find faith.

Wednesday 14 April

I played for Post Office FC tonight against Malton. I've lost it. I stretched every sinew to bomb up and down the left wing to feed our front two. My efforts felt pathetic and futile. I was surrounded by faster, sprightlier and spottier players who haven't yet left their teens. I detected snorts of derision as they whipped past me. I resigned myself to just trying to win throw-ins. How the average fall! I've treasured playing this game with blokes like these. Wellsy popped up in the last minute to score a brilliant winner. What a rush of sheer joy it was to dive on him in celebration.

I've received another email from the Oasis documentary team. They want to film me and a congregation singing one of Noel's songs during a Sunday service. Even I would struggle to make that happen. No church I know would let me sandwich 'Thine be the Glory' between 'Cigarettes and Alcohol' and 'Rock and Roll Star'. Or would they? I'll ask around.

We find out if the IVF has worked tomorrow. Anna is convinced that she's not pregnant. I walked the streets for a while trying to prepare myself for the worst. The music of the Eels was my soundtrack. These sad but hopeful songs were so fitting. I went past West Bank Park and saw Aunty Lynne, Ally, Mum, Grandma, Jo, Beck, Lorrie and the babies by the picnic tables. They looked sad too. I joined them and we sat in numbed silence. Nothing needed to be said. I stopped off at my sister's house for a nervous poo. Amy was fuming.

I've come to bed early. Tomorrow can't come soon enough. This weight needs lifting from our marriage one way or another. Anna is next to me. She's pretending to be asleep, I think. Waiting. Is our child growing inside her?

Thursday 15 April

Anna is five weeks' pregnant. Incredible! After years of heartache, three rounds of IVF and a very sad wife, a baby is now growing inside Anna. Our baby! Thank you, God! We're still coming to terms with it. It's the fulfilment of so much prayer from so many different people. I know there's a long way to go before we hold our son or daughter in our arms, but wow! It's even more remarkable given that he or she has been created from one of my old frozen sperm. It proves that there's always hope. Anna's face is a picture of sheer, unadulterated joy. I keep catching myself breaking out into one of those stupid, soppy smiles.

The events of this morning are vivid. We arrived at Seacroft Hospital for 10 a.m., heavy of heart, not daring to dream. Anna was convinced that her period was imminent. A nurse with a kind face called Jane ushered us into a side room. She disappeared with Anna's urine sample. We clung onto each other, bracing ourselves for bad news. Jane returned, placed a hand on each of our shoulders, looked deep into Anna's eyes, and said the four most glorious words of our lives: 'Congratulations – you are pregnant!' Anna cried out, *'Really?!'* I may have sworn.

Jane told us that she was on a roll – it was the fourth positive result she'd given to a couple that morning. She has the best job and worst job in the world. We were shown the pregnancy test and there, unmistakably, was the magical pink line. We got home and did another test just to be sure – there was the pink line again! And then we did it again. And again. And again. Our thirst to see the pink line would not be sated! It turns out that Anna had planned to do a test at home last night to put herself out of the misery. But then in a quiet moment with God, she read this in her Bible: 'Be still and know that I am God.'

Anna called her mum in the hospital car park and wept big, happy tears. Our parents have lived this pain with us. What a privilege to now share our joy with them. We decided to share our news with the world at this early stage because so many were aware of our situation. And, as Anna pointed out, I can't ever keep my mouth shut. Some cried when we told them (even Lee, which surprised me). Some said they knew this would happen (like Grandma). Others just screamed down the phone (my sister). My

Cranmer mates were ecstatic. Their prayers and anointing that special night in the chapel was a significant moment. They prayed in real faith when I was low on it. Archbishop Sentamu was buzzing when he heard. We were brought down to earth a bit tonight when Anna experienced some abdominal pain. We've just got to trust God now. He has brought us this far. My wife is five weeks' pregnant!

Friday 16 April

I got up at 5 a.m. to pray and read the Bible. Sleep was impossible after our big news. It was a special few hours. I felt as fresh as a young salmon by the end of it. My prayer remains the same: to be just a bit more like Jesus every day. I checked with Anna every few minutes that her insides were free of pain and ache. Only eight more months of worry to go.

Saturday 17 April

I give thanks for afternoons like this with Dad. There's no one I'd rather be in the Swan with to watch the footy results come in. His interest is infectious. He made me care passionately for Rochdale who were promoted for the first time in 40 years. I crave more times like this with Dad. But he can never sustain it. It can only ever be a relationship of fleeting moments and thrilling but short-lived encounters. Usually in bars. I can't moan. I'd rather have an up-and-down dad than no dad.

I played an 11-a-side game for St Paul's Church against a bunch of lawyers this morning. One of our lads suffered a bad leg break. There was an audible, sickening crack when he went in for a tackle on the keeper. He went down, screaming: 'It's broken! I've broken my leg! It's gone, it's broken!' Some of the guys thought he was joking but I knew different. I tried to comfort him and make him laugh before the paramedics arrived. They administered gas and air. He went from crying with pain to crying with laughter. I told him that I didn't think my jokes were that funny.

Monday 19 April

It's strange being back at Cranmer knowing that Anna is pregnant at home. Everyone is encouraged that our prayers have been answered. It's nice for a group of trainee vicars to be reminded that God actually intervenes sometimes when we ask him to. We now have a two-week teaching block on sex and gender. It could be an incendiary topic in an environment like this. I'm determined not to light any fuses, I've decided to keep my own counsel and stay quiet for the whole two weeks. With topics like homosexuality, women in leadership and why blokes hate going to church on the agenda, it won't be easy. There are times to be an outspoken, clownish loudmouth. This isn't one of them.

Tuesday 20 April

My self-induced sex and gender silence has been too deafening for some. I can't win. I'm determined not to become embroiled in a pointless row. This is not the module to shoot from the hip. We can resolve nothing here, but we have the potential to cause lasting division if we're not careful. I'm starting to sound like Kofi Annan from the UN.

We were split into mixed groups. I ended up with two middle-aged Methodist students, Aidan and a few others. Our first task was genuinely shocking. With little drama or fuss, we were asked to put in order of extremity a list of every sexual activity we could think of. The sheet had 'holding hands' at the bottom and 'full penetrative sex' at the top. 'Just fill in the blanks!' the session leader trilled. The point of it was to take away the fear factor when talking about sex in our parishes. It may have scarred me for life. When I enrolled at Cranmer, I couldn't have imagined that I'd be required to discuss the relative severity of dry humping, fellatio and anal sex. It was like playing an explicit game of Top Trumps.

Some of the class enjoyed the exercise a bit *too* much. Others became frenzied doodlers, refusing to look up, pretending it wasn't happening. One of the Methodist students was virtually rocking back and forth with her thumb in, whispering 'take me to a happy place'. I only had one beef with our group's sex list: dry humping is way more serious than neck nuzzling.

Wednesday 21 April

Jason is back. What a relief. He's on the mend at last. His tutors have ordered him to take it easy and forget about writing essays for now. Every cloud and all that. Aidan was very down at Morning Glory. Claire has suffered another bout of illness, which makes the likelihood of them being allowed to have kids extremely unlikely. They're now trying to get their heads round the possibility of adoption.

Thursday 22 April

Conflict follows me around like the smell of fags on an old pair of jeans. I somehow managed to have bust-ups with two Morning Glory members today. Aidan was understandable. It would be an exceptional day if we didn't have some kind of verbal spat. But Rob Lee? It shouldn't be possible. It's like falling out with Mother Teresa, the Dalai Lama and Mary Poppins all rolled into one.

Aidan and I had gone for it in the common room when he accused me of being too critical about Cranmer. He'd walked in on me venting my spleen about some of our lectures needing to be more relentless in applying to real life. Same rant, different day. Aidan is an intellectual snob at times. I guess he'd accuse me of being boorish, impatient and insensitive. Ironically, I'm learning more from our fractious relationship about God, myself and the joy and struggles of Christian community than anything else.

My row with Rob came about after a port-fuelled flower arranging session. I accused him of being like one of the pigs from *Animal Farm* because of the way I sometimes see him conforming to the stuffy, rigid ways of the Church of England. It was out of order. It wasn't true. Rob just looked at me wearily before sloping off to bed. I'll need to put some more humble pie in the oven tomorrow.

The flower arranging itself was a blast. Jason and I wanted to honour our commitment to go on the college rota after being critical of it within earshot of some practitioners. Lubricated by port, brie and crisps, the night was a triumph. Who knew that arranging flowers could be so sociable and therapeutic? The conversation was deep, honest and deliciously indiscreet. My favourite kind.

Friday 23 April

More revelations in sex and gender. Today we were given a breakdown of the basics of sex therapy. I now know more than I ever wanted to about issues surrounding orgasms, clitorises and necrophilia. Too much information!

Anna has discovered that this is the day in the pregnancy cycle when our baby is supposed to generate a heartbeat. We went to Mum's for prayer. It's all getting very real. Anna tried to begin the conversation about how the baby will change things. I couldn't have it. It's too early. There's too much that could go wrong. I just want to know if we've got a heartbeat at the moment.

Saturday 24 April

Anna is full of fear and dread. I wish she could just enjoy the experience of being pregnant. It's easier said than done. We're both completely neurotic that something inside her is going wrong. Every time her stomach gurgles I go into a blind panic and want to take her to A and E.

Sunday 25 April

Anna brought me tea and crumpets in bed this morning. Shouldn't I be doing that kind of thing for her?

Tuesday 27 April

It's quite a personal achievement that I've not yet uttered a single word of wisdom, an amusing quip, or an impassioned rant to the rest of the class during our sex and gender module. I feel a new-found affinity to introverts. It's interesting what you notice when you just watch and listen. My colleagues have been noticeably careful in their musings. They've largely kept their own counsel on issues such as homosexuality and sex before marriage. Not causing offence is very important to people here. As I said to the lads afterwards: 'It's so PC in here that we should be working for Microsoft!'

The sessions took a bizarre twist this afternoon. Our task was to rate out of ten what we thought our desirability was to the opposite sex. It was the lecturer's way of preparing us for the bombshell claim that when we are ordained we could add 5 to that figure. What?! In other words we become 50 per cent more sexually desirable once we have a dog collar on. Some of the class looked a little too pleased with the revelation.

Thursday 29 April

The issue of homosexuality finally raised its head in sex and gender today. It was interesting to observe that among the different theological traditions represented in the class, each one of them thinks that there is an inherent bias towards their theological opposites. So the liberals believe there is an evangelical church bias towards the view that homosexuality is wrong. The more conservative evangelicals claim there is a growing liberal culture within the Anglican tradition and something of an 'anything goes' mentality. The lecturers fudged the session, but I don't blame them. Long-held theological and moral beliefs don't change after a classroom bust-up. People just get upset.

There was still a simmering tension throughout the session as folk desperately tried to keep a dignified silence. It ended with the same reflection that all difficult ethical issues and debates seem to conclude with: it's all part of 'God's mystery'. I'm getting tired of hearing that.

The producers of the Oasis documentary now want me to talk about the song 'Let There Be Love'. I've been given permission to use the college chapel to do the filming.

My tutor Stuart gave me a mild telling-off this afternoon. He pinpointed two recent occasions when he felt I'd spoken out of turn at college. (Only two?) The first was when I asked the head of Traidcraft in a lecture why fair trade tea bags always tasted dodgy. The second was when I told a random, hirsute gentleman who was visiting college that he had a great beard and looked like a bishop I know. Fair enough. I'm still learning to stop the things that pop into my head coming out of my mouth.

Friday 30 April

I sent one of the lads a card to encourage him about the dignified way he has carried himself these past two weeks in sex and gender. I've begun to appreciate how difficult life must be for a gay Christian at college. It really can't be easy.

Today's last session was on family life. No one seemed to have much positive to say about it – or positive experiences of it. How sad. Our lecturer gave a depressing account from the Bible. He's clearly a brilliant man, but I wish he'd get off the fence occasionally. In the later session, it was claimed that the woman caught in adultery from the Gospel of John had not committed adultery at all. It was an interesting, feminist perspective but seemed to me to devalue Christ's central message of grace and reconciliation. I despair at theological study sometimes. Now even one of my most treasured gospel stories might not be true. Thanks for that.

Anna and I saw Peter Kay in Manchester tonight. I needed a few laughs.

Wednesday 5 May

We find out if everything is as it should be with our baby tomorrow. Anna keeps punishing herself by logging onto the IVF internet forums. No one seems to post good news. It's all complications and tragic tales. She's now banned from these sites.

Aunty Lynne's specialist has said that surgery is not out of the question following her course of chemotherapy. We're staying positive.

Thursday 6 May

We're having twins! Twins! Somehow my pathetic frozen sperm have produced two of the little blighters! What a day. I got up at 6 a.m. to pray, focus and vote. We drove to Seacroft Hospital in nervous silence. We've grown to hate that journey. George, our favourite nurse, called us up from that anxious waiting room pretty quickly. A probe-type thing was inserted into Anna as she lay on the bed. Almost immediately George made some positive noises and said she'd found a heartbeat. We could see it on the monitor flickering like an asteroid from a 1980s arcade game. Then she asked how many embryos had been put back in. We told her two. George then just blurted out: 'Oh look, another one!' Two heartbeats! There they were, flashing side by side on the screen. We didn't have any words to convey the shock and joy of that moment. It was wildest dream territory. Two babies are actually alive and growing inside my wife right at this moment.

George talked us through the next steps but I wasn't listening. I was thinking about that doctor who told me on the phone that if he was a betting man he wouldn't put money on me ever becoming a father. Nothing is impossible with God. He has blessed us beyond our most optimistic hopes. Prayer actually works! George gave us photos of our children to take home. *Our children.* Plural. Wow!

We walked out of the hospital desperate to tell the whole world. Anna wanted to tell her mum first in person. We drove back in numbed silence, soaking in the enormity of the news. We tricked our mums by showing them one photo before I came in with the second one. My favourite phone call was to Martin – the man who made it possible. 'You've paid for two babies,' I told him. I texted all our family and friends with the words: 'It's twins! Oh crap!' I went for a run to clear my head before going round to tell Dad and Maggie. He cracked open a bottle of champagne to celebrate. My head was unclear again within the hour. Somehow in all the excitement I managed to short-circuit their electrics after falling into their living room lamp.

Attempting to sleep is futile. It's looking likely that I'll be the father of two children. Lord have mercy on us all!

Friday 7 May

I woke up with a sore head but a bursting heart. I'm going to be a dad to twins. Ouch! Anna says she feels pregnant now. Her only complaint is that her boobs are sore. Physically, I've never been more attracted to Anna. Within seconds of us getting round to her mum's they were discussing which pushchair to buy and possible names. Anna deserves this. After years of enduring endless baby talk she can finally join in. What a gift.

Saturday 8 May

Big study day. I'm writing an essay on male spirituality, and, more specifically, why so many men hate going to church. How can the church be more effective at reaching out to them? Blokes fascinate me. We are complex creatures. Generally speaking, the men I interact with fall into two categories. There's the sensitive types who are in touch with their feminine sides. They don't have an issue expressing how they feel. Then – more commonly – there's the practical, no-nonsense type of blokes who are perhaps, on the surface, more closed books emotionally. They're happy to talk football, cars and power tools, but struggle with anything deeper.

A writer called James Nelson has an interesting theory. He reckons that men should regain an 'intimate connection' between their spirituality and sexuality. Apparently we are often too hung up – and often slaves to – our 'phallic' side, which is manifested by us doing, producing or performing. Nelson argues that we also need to incorporate our 'penis side' which is manifested by us feeling, relaxing and expressing emotion. The phallus and penis – our hard and soft sides – can work together to get us closer to God.

Jesus, of course, was not afraid to show his hard and soft sides. He was a carpenter who drove the traders from the temple but also cried openly at the death of his friend Lazarus. Nelson says that men need to learn to cry 'tears of the penis'. I'm trying to imagine sharing these revelations with the Post Office footy lads. I can't.

I've just tried in vain to get Anna interested in my phallic side. She grunted and turned over. Fair enough.

Sunday 9 May

Anna was an emotional wreck all day. I hated leaving her to come back to Durham. She clung to me and wept. Her worries are many and varied. She fears I'll miss the babies being born. She is fretting about where we'll end up after Cranmer. I think they call this the 'nesting' instinct kicking in.

Aidan preached without notes at church tonight. He was brilliant. Git.

Tuesday 11 May

Joel Wood leaned over to me during tonight's college Communion. He blazed his eyes into mine and whispered: 'Never get out of the ring, Woody. Never get out of the ring.' I'm not entirely sure what he meant, but it gave me goosebumps.

Wednesday 12 May

I basked in the intimacy of a holy moment tonight. I was overcome by a thankfulness to God. Prayed that I might truly live a life of service to others. A fresh blast of priestly calling rattled and stirred me. The enormity of what God was asking me to do and who he was asking me to be hit me afresh. I committed to him that if I'm doing it and being it then it's with two feet in. No holding back. No fear.

I read an article in *The Times* recently about a vicar who was walking along the street in a dodgy part of London's East End. A destitute woman begged him for food and shelter. He did what he could, but was determined to provide more permanent help. His clergy colleagues dismissed his dream as pointless folly. The vicar didn't listen. He went on to pioneer a shelter in his parish which has since flourished. I want to be a priest like that. One who dreams crazy dreams and makes them happen. A priest who doesn't listen to those who say it can't be done. Or that it shouldn't be done. Show me the way, Lord.

Rhys Thomas shared a stinker of a Bible verse this morning from Ephesians 3.10. It had us all floundering. 'His intent was that now, through the church, the manifold wisdom of God should be made known to the rulers and authorities in the heavenly realms.' No one seems to have a clue what or who it's on about. Is it referring to angels in the heavenly realms? How do we make God's wisdom known to them? Surely they know him already because they're up there with him? Even Rob Lee was baffled and he knows *everything*.

Anna went into meltdown as we chatted on Skype tonight. Between snotty sobs, she wailed: 'Will I be a good enough mum?'

Thursday 13 May

I've been given a high mark for my assessed sermon on church unity. Praise from our principal, David, has lifted me into the clouds somewhere. He is that rare breed of academic who is always the cleverest guy in the room, but also the most humble. He's able to communicate the Christian faith in a way that's relevant, engaging and inspiring. So for him to say that my sermon was 'outstanding' is special. David's sidekick, our brilliant preaching tutor, Kate, said I just need to be careful that my 'spontaneous humour moments' don't get out of hand or draw attention away from God. That's like asking a Tourette's sufferer not to swear.

Friday 14 May

Driving back to York, I received the worst possible text from Anna. It said, simply: 'I've started bleeding a bit.' I succumbed to an awful dread. My imagination whipped me into a frenzy of worst possible scenarios. By the time I pulled into Glebe Avenue, I was picturing Anna slumped over on a bloodied bathroom floor, dead-eyed and wailing like one of those grieving mothers from the Gaza Strip. In reality, though, all was well. Of course it was. I demanded detailed information about how much she'd bled and what we could do about it. We later discovered that many women experience 'spotting' during pregnancy. It had stopped by late afternoon. I can't go on like this. I'm living in constant fear that all will be lost.

Sunday 16 May

I skipped church this morning and enjoyed an act of worship in our conservatory. I meditated on Psalm 51. It's King David's great prayer of repentance. It struck me reading it that, above all else, God wants us to be honest with him. To lay bare our innermost feelings, desires and weaknesses. Verse 6 spoke to me in particular: 'surely you desire truth in the inner parts'. After a glorious egg sandwich, Anna followed me upstairs for a 'snooze'. We both knew the score. I loved it. All three minutes of it. Anna is becoming deliciously curvy. Her body is transforming into a feeding machine. We later watched York City get stuffed 3–1 by Oxford in the Division Two play-offs. More days like this, please.

Wednesday 19 May

I received a card from Anna. It shows two women in a supermarket inspecting bottles of wine. One is thinking: 'Hmmm, delicate top notes of citrus and blackberry with a cheeky hint of vanilla on the afterburn. Delightful.' The other woman is thinking: 'Ah, three for ten pounds. Intriguing.' She knows me.

Joel and I filmed our contribution to the Oasis documentary in the chapel today. We wore black robes and spoke in front of the big crucifix to give it that trainee vicar vibe. It was all going well until Joel blurted out: 'Liam and Noel are like prophets.' I'm sure that's the bit they'll use. He could get us both fired for heresy! Prophets, no. Rock gods, yes.

Thursday 20 May

My assessed pastoral interview has received some wonderfully peculiar feedback. It was the one where I invited the lonely wife of the abusive alcoholic down the pub. In his written feedback, my tutor wrote that I'd failed to pick up on the 'sexual undertones' apparent during the interview. What?! Apparently the actress lady had reported that if I'm not careful, some women I encounter in a ministerial setting will 'fall in love' with me. Surely it would be more worrying if I had picked up on these so-called sexual undertones? It wasn't as if she was looking at me longingly or suggestively. I would have noticed. She was a crying mess of bubble and snot. And she's in her mid-60s – at least. It couldn't have been less sexy if we were both sat in a bath of cold baked beans. I'm actually very happy that I didn't notice these alleged undertones. How I'll avoid women falling in love with me when I become a reverend is another matter. Ask them to babysit, perhaps?

Friday 21 May

Passions were stirred and fires stoked in our diversity seminar today. We debated the view that Christianity – by its very nature – is not 'fair'. The point was made that Christians don't believe in pure equality because of the central claim that the only way to God in heaven is through Jesus Christ. Before long, the classroom echoed to the sound of theological colours being pinned to the mast. We are a wonderful, incendiary mix of woolly, anything goes liberals; black-and-white, frothing conservative evangelicals and classic central Anglican fence-sitters. I'm still working out which theological position I call home.

In a vociferous celebration of our diversity, Neil and Joel really went at it. Neil argued that as church leaders we should relentlessly aspire to total equality, no matter what the circumstances. Joel asked how this would work with paedophiles and murderers. Should they be given the same rights and privileges in a church setting as everyone else? Things got louder and fingers more pointed from that moment on.

Just when things seemed to be calming down, Joel waded in with the view that the Royal Family are the key to the next phase of Christendom. Boom – we were off again! At the end of the lesson we all discovered that someone had anonymously left a Curly Wurly in our pigeon holes. Great timing. As we chomped and chewed, we decided we loved each other really. There's real power in a free Curly Wurly.

Saturday 22 May

I joined my mate Pete's band onstage for the end of their set at Anne's 50th birthday party. She's a precious friend to us. I nervously strummed along to 'I Am the Walrus' and 'She's Electric'. Why couldn't this have been my calling?

Monday 24 May

A visiting US professor of astronomy blew my mind as well as opened it during his lecture tonight. How refreshing to hear staggering revelations about the enormity and complexity of the universe from such a committed Christian. Who says theology and science don't mix? He was the guest of our principal, David, who is himself one of the country's most respected cosmologists. Hearing people of immense intellect declare their faith within the context of the most complex science helps my faith. Somehow I feel more secure knowing that they believe too.

The professor gave us a whirlwind tour of the universe to highlight just how incomprehensibly vast it is. He took us as far as the Hubble telescopes can reach – all the way to quasars. They're stars that existed billions of years ago, apparently. We were treated to stunning PowerPoint images of planets, dust clouds, red stars, supermassive black holes and colliding stars. In the Q and A, I asked if he thought God had created life elsewhere. He said – given the enormity of the universe – that it would be strange if there was no life elsewhere.

The professor's description of the depth of God's love for us in the context of the vast universe was profoundly moving. Jesus could have stopped time and space with the flick of his fingers, yet he chose to stay and die in terrible pain so that we might live. Words can't express the enormity of a love like that.

Paul Bromley was on hilarious form this morning. I picked him up from Scotch Corner and he immediately broke into his Stephen Hawking voice. Later on in lectures we drew inappropriate doodles. It's not good. I'm reliving my early teens. We're on a four-day placement together from tomorrow at a nearby primary school. Lord, help them.

Tuesday 25 May

It was the worst possible start for Paul and me on our primary school placement. A flatulent six-year-old girl let rip during our first RE lesson. How anything so aggressively cacophonous could come out of one so young and small is beyond me. I made the huge tactical error of catching Paul's eye. That was it. We both lost it completely. Tears rolled down our cheeks. I frantically tried to conjure up sad, horrible thoughts in an effort to stop the flow of uncontrollable hysterics. Paul rubbed his eyes furiously. I dread to think how unprofessional we must have looked. We're like *Beavis and Butt-head* with a faith. The irony that it's the school's 'fun week' wasn't lost on us.

Wednesday 26 May

I'm loving schools week. I bonded with the class clown in Mrs Grayson's form. Making his mates laugh and keeping abreast of the football transfer market is all Lewis seems to care about. It was like talking to my ten-year-old self.

Thursday 27 May

One of the teachers I spent the morning with was overcome with tears at break time. It turns out that her little niece will lose her eye after walking into a tree branch. Life makes no sense to me sometimes.

At the post-lunch register time Miss Warne put me on the naughty board for talking. The kids loved it. One of them blurted out: 'Are you Miss Warne's boyfriend?' Awkward. Earlier a little lad called me 'Mr Big Nose'. He later came over in tears with a letter of apology addressed to 'Mr Woodcuts'. Paul and I left cards and chocolates for the staff before we said our goodbyes. Great week.

Sunday 30 May

In preparation for her chemotherapy, Aunty Lynne has been shopping for a wig. Becky said it looks just like her normal hair. I keep hoping and praying that all will be well.

I visited a local charismatic church this morning. I craved something a bit more happy clappy. My soul needed a joy injection after the drudgery of Morning Prayer. Unfortunately the sermon was an absolute motorway pile-up. The preacher didn't inspire confidence when his opening gambit was all about how nervous he felt. 'I nearly chickened out of doing this last night,' he told us. It got worse. The poor guy paced around the stage with a haunted expression on his face, mumbling seemingly random thoughts and reflections. I think – but it's only a guess – that he was trying to communicate something about us taking personal responsibility. He referred to the Book of Ruth a bit and a 'triangle matrix' to explain our relationship between God, the Church and the world. Then he suddenly remembered he wanted to use the Good Samaritan as an illustration but couldn't remember why. It felt like an eternity as he frantically tried to recall it. He seemed close to walking off. The communal relief when he finally finished was palpable. I nearly gave him a clap. It reminded me of Rowan Atkinson conducting that wedding ceremony in *Four Weddings and a Funeral*.

Monday 31 May

I've decided on a boy's name: Freddie Romero. I love it. Anna still needs convincing, though. It came to me in the shower while thinking of men who inspired me. Oscar Romero and Freddie Flintoff – what a combination! They're fine men for Woody Junior to seek to emulate. Archbishop Romero, a courageous man of faith, hero of the poor and oppressed. Martyred in cold blood while presiding at Holy Communion by gunmen loyal to San Salvador's vicious dictator. And Freddie – lion-hearted Ashes legend (and the name of Anna's late grandpa). Sorted.

Tuesday 1 June

I met Joel Wood in Durham Cathedral's café to tell him about my fear of dogs. It's time I was free of it. Every nightmare I wake from finds me running from or being chewed by some big-jawed mutt. I still have to cross the road if one is coming the other way.

Joel reassured me that God's love leaves no place for such fear to flourish in my life. He became excited at the idea of praying about it by the sacred tomb of St Cuthbert. This Celtic saint was a spiritual titan apparently. He's one of Joel's heroes. I wasn't thrilled with the idea. The tomb is one of the cathedral's major draws. Tourists were swarming all around it. Joel doesn't do embarrassment, though.

We squeezed past them and knelt down at the foot of the tomb. He laid his hand on my back and asked God to lift my fear. After a while a wonderful peace came over me. It wasn't weird or exaggerated. It felt real and lovely. Like Jesus was kneeling right there with us. When we opened our eyes a special hush had descended over the spot. The cameras had stopped clicking. A foreign tourist had knelt down beside us to pray. I felt a real sense of release. That is right up until we walked back to college by the river. A black dog suddenly jumped out in front of us. It was big and boisterous. Was this my big test? If it was, I failed. Big time. I let out a pathetic scream and hid behind Joel, clutching onto his unfeasibly long trouser leg like a cowardly ten-year-old. He looked down at me with such understanding and compassion. He is my St Cuthbert.

Wednesday 2 June

The entire Cranmer posse piled onto buses for a day of prayer and reflection on Holy Island. I spent two hours sat on the rock where I proposed to Anna. The sun broke through the clouds and shone on my face. What a contrast to that day in 2004. Rain lashed down as she reluctantly agreed to crouch on the rock for the big moment. I remember she looked ridiculously cute with her hood up. I pulled out the mini bottle of Moet from my rucksack and got down on one knee. It was the wettest proposal ever. Perhaps it was a portent of things to come. Our marriage is always in the extreme of sunshine or storm. Peace or chaos. Laughter or shouts. Rarely is it ever dull or overcast. That's how we roll.

I read Bede's *Life of St Cuthbert* as I sat there, imagining him walking around the island. Cuthbert is fast becoming one of my Christian heroes. He was the first pioneer. He is the template for what a priest should be like. As Bede writes:

He [St Cuthbert] made a point of searching out those steep rugged places in the hills which other preachers dreaded to visit because of their poverty and squalor. This, to him, was a labour of love. He was so keen to preach that sometimes he would be away for a whole week or a fortnight, or even a month, living with rough hill folk, preaching and calling them heavenwards by his example.

Every one of us about to take holy orders, every important God person in a pointy hat and fancy robes should take heed: *it's about the people.* Cuthbert's prayer life was extraordinary. He'd spend whole nights praying while up to his neck in freezing sea water. He felt it would keep him more alert and attentive to God. Astonishing. Holy Island is often described as a 'thin place'. That it is somehow closer to God because of the amount of prayer that has gone on there. I agree. Special times.

It was our last Morning Glory meeting of the college year this morning. Jason challenged me that I was too aloof and didn't 'let him in'. He wants us to be closer friends. I'll try.

Tuesday 8 June

We've made it to twelve weeks. Anna is huge already. Her tummy is a thing of beauty. I can't stop stroking it and putting my ear to it. The pregnancy experts we've read online say that reaching this milestone is extremely significant. The chances of miscarriage go right down. I love the opinion of experts when it's good news. One of the unfortunate side-effects is Anna's snoring. I may as well be lying next to an asthmatic boar. So, so loud. I'm daring to dream now that this might actually happen.

I've got to preach about hell this Sunday at my new placement church. Not the greatest way to ingratiate myself with these people. It's no one's favourite subject.

Wednesday 9 June

I reluctantly made an appearance at a morning ecumenical prayer meeting for church leaders. It's not for me really. The people are lovely but I always feel a bit awkward and out of place at such gatherings. The demographic is predominantly late middle-aged males with beards. Lots and lots of beards. It's dominated by charismatic types who seem to love the sound of their own prayers. I wonder sometimes if God gets weary of these wordy intercessions. Perhaps he'd prefer us to shut up and listen to what he has to say?

Friday 11 June

The vicar at my latest placement church goes door knocking around his parish every Friday afternoon. It's old school but seems to work. He has a lovely relaxed manner. The dog collar works wonders. I took on a few streets with him round the local council estate. It was an eye-opener. So many people we spoke to don't even know what the church is *for*.

My worst fear was realized at the first door I knocked on. A dog with a baritone bark. It sounded as big as a horse. The family were poor. They thought I was there to sell them insurance. I tried to sell them the idea of church. It wasn't successful. At the next house the guy had very few teeth. Before long he was telling me about his difficult relationship with his stepson. I then got talking to a pram-pushing young father on the street. His other kids were baptized at the church a few years ago but they didn't return. They'd enjoyed the singing, though. I invited him back – with the promise that his sons would be well looked after for an hour. I felt like a salesman promising the offer of free childcare if he signed on the dotted line and came to church.

My last and most significant encounter was with a bin man called Brian. He was sat in a deckchair in his front garden flanked by a huge, sinister-looking friend. They both wore stained white vests. Brian was openly hostile at first. He shouted at me that the church was a disgrace for refusing to baptize his stepdaughter's baby. Eventually I persuaded him to explain what happened. He offered me a deckchair and a can. It was a wonderful experience. Brian told me all about his life as a bin man and the joys and pain of his family. I asked what he wanted from his local vicar. Perhaps Brian's view about church and Christianity might be more positive now. I've made arrangements for his stepdaughter's baby to get baptized.

Saturday 12 June

How did I end up watching the England game with Anna and her mum? It was really tense. Not that they were remotely interested. At a crucial point in the match, I suddenly became aware that they were talking excitedly across me about an amazing bargain they'd noticed at Asda. I silently fumed. If it was *Corrie* there'd be hell on.

Sunday 13 June

Joel and I featured in the Oasis documentary tonight on Channel 4. It was called *What's Your Story?* Fans from all over the world talked about what the band means to them. One guy was a Liam impersonator from Italy. Another bloke revealed that their music literally saved his life. Suddenly we popped up on screen sat in front of the chapel cross dressed in our black robes. As predicted, they edited Joel so all he said was, 'They are prophets.' It featured me reading out the lyrics to 'Let There Be Love' before cutting into the song itself with footage of them playing live. Despite the late hour, friends and family texted to say they'd seen it. Uncle Mike said it made him cry! I can only hope Noel was watching.

Tuesday 15 June

The Bishop of Hull called me out of the blue tonight. It felt significant. He wanted to sound me out about a potential curacy at Holy Trinity Church in Hull city centre. I've never heard of the place. Apparently it's the largest parish church building in England. William Wilberforce was baptized there. Despite being Hull's civic church, it's on its knees financially and in terms of numbers and outreach. Worship-wise it's very traditional, with robes and a choir. The liturgy probably goes on for days.

I said I wanted a challenge. Bishop Richard said a new vicar – Neal Barnes – is about to start there. He's highly thought of. They're looking for a pioneer minister to work with him. Interesting. I told him that the big issue could be Anna. She is adamant that we won't leave York. I tentatively mentioned it to her 'in passing' to gauge the reaction. It could have been worse. The initial wall of ice thawed ever so slightly as we talked about how it could work. The crucial sticking point for me is whether I could work with Neal. Is he robust and releasing enough to cope with me? I'll research him and pray about it. If God wants us in Hull then it will happen.

I met Helena for coffee to reminisce about our days working together at St Paul's. There was an excruciating moment when I saw an old guy from my placement church in the queue to pay. From his gestures I thought he had bought our drinks. He hadn't. I kept thanking him really loudly. He just looked at me with a puzzled expression. Then the waitress handed me our bill. How embarrassing.

Sunday 20 June

My hell sermon has received positive feedback from my placement vicar. I'm passionate that preaching should always stir our senses – laughter, anger, tears, whatever. But it must stir something, anything in fact. If our hearers are bored and disengaged we're not doing it properly. My preaching mantra is this: if I don't feel it, I can't preach it. We'll see where that gets me.

Monday 21 June

It was a surreal moment seeing the twins move on screen during the ultrasound. Babies we'd made were alive and wriggling. They were our babies! We'd waited so long for that moment it felt like a bit of an anti-climax. There was a horrible minute or so when the nurse had to check everything was OK before letting us see the images. As she glided the sensor around Anna's jellied belly for signs of life, I studied her face intently for signs of concern. It was like watching the cabin crew during flight turbulence. All was well, though. Our babies are alive, breathing and formed! Anna cried tears of joy.

Saturday 26 June

Pete Hale and I walked 25 miles up the three Yorkshire peaks, Pen Y Ghent, Wernside and Ingleborough, in 8 hours, 55 minutes. I'm chuffed with that. We didn't have a map, or much kit, but we went for it anyway. Loads of people were doing it for charity. I got a text from Jason half way up one of the peaks to say Ruth had given birth to Hannah Louise. Wonderful. Walking downhill was a killer on the knees. We kept seeing the bloke who plays Eric Pollard from *Emmerdale.* He lapped up the attention. I forced Pete to run the last mile or so with me in order to break our sub-nine-hour target. Our first pint in the pub in Horton was joy itself.

Monday 28 June

I'm helping a church in York with their communications as part of a mini-placement. I got onto the subject of healing with a lovely lady there. She told me that her friend had been suffering from painful verrucas so she offered to pray. 'As I was praying at her feet I felt God saying that I should spit on the verrucas,' she went on. 'Wow, what happened – did it work?' I asked, expectantly. 'Not in the slightest!' she replied, exploding into a laughing fit.

Anna and I attended the second session of the marriage course at St Paul's tonight. I moaned about having to miss the football. She wasn't impressed. The session's theme was forgiveness. How appropriate.

Thursday 1 July

I'm reading *Love in the Time of Cholera* by Gabriel García Márquez. The writing has a wonderful poetry and rhythm to it.

I've bought the *Sun* every day this week to keep in touch with what's getting the masses talking. It has all been England World Cup flops, Kelly Brook on jet skis and twins being mauled by foxes. People are always 'outraged' in the tabloid world. I watched *Rev* for the first time. It was a pleasant surprise. The Revd Adam Smallbone has a genuine humanity and warmth that I related to. In the opening scene, he invites his small congregation back to the vicarage for 'a glass of something cold'. It cuts to the morning after with Adam and his wife in bed with stinking hangovers. Bottles and mess are strewn everywhere. Brilliant. Anna and I go to Tenerife tomorrow for what we hope is our last holiday as a childless couple.

Friday 2 July

I blended in at Leeds Bradford Airport by settling down in the bar with a lager and a copy of the *Sun*. It was 7 a.m. Our flight was dominated by a raucous, intimidating stag-do from Bradford. The flight attendants gave each other a despairing look as they boarded. The lads were clearly on a mission to get annihilated before they even reached Tenerife. We'd barely left the ground when other passengers began to complain about their swearing and lewd stories. The captain came over on the tannoy to appeal for calm. When we eventually landed, one of the stags climbed onto the moving luggage carousel. He was dragged off by security to the cheers of 30 plastered Bradfordians.

Our apartment has a sea view. That makes me very, very happy.

Saturday 3 July

Sea views fill me with a child-like wonder. I try to imagine where the different shipping vessels are heading to and the purpose of their voyage. I'm literally turning into my dad.

We've received some more extraordinary news from our IVF benefactor. Martin texted to say he is giving us a further £2,000 because 'twins are expensive'. Is there no limit to this man's generosity? He has inspired us to rethink how we view money and giving. We want to live with his spirit of generosity. Martin acts like it's not his money. Like he's just looking after it for God. Like he's on a never-ending quest to see who he can help with it.

A local barber has massacred my hair. His English wasn't brilliant. He clearly didn't understand what I wanted. Now I have a 1989-inspired flat top. I look like Drago from *Rocky IV.*

Sunday 4 July

I've received my latest church placement report. It's glowing. The vicar's one criticism is that people may find me 'exhausting'.

Anna and I had an entertaining evening at a pizza restaurant with a comedian for a waiter and a musician in love with Dire Straits.

Monday 5 July

Ian called to say that Lisa's Uncle Bob has died. He's Sarah Bulmer's dad. *The* Sarah Bulmer. The Sarah Bulmer who sent my 17-year-old heart into a thumping, mushy mess when we worked weekends together at the Posthouse. I was a porter. She was a chambermaid – and all I wanted in a woman back then, though we never quite made it romantically. Not after she snogged Glen Flanagan in Silks on that staff night out. Anyway, in a strange set of circumstances, the family have asked me to take Bob's funeral at York Crematorium. It would be my first one. What a privilege. I just need to find out what you actually do and say. This vicar stuff is getting a bit too real.

I'm reading another Maigret novel. The best bits are always when he's in a bar pondering his latest case. Simenon puts us right there with him. Every sip of wine, every pull on his pipe, becomes more compelling than the murder itself.

Tuesday 6 July

Our waiter undercharged us for our seafood risotto and half carafe of wine in the restaurant tonight. We owned up. It felt good to be good.

Wednesday 7 July

Tenerife's capital, Santa Cruz, was an unexpected delight as I took refuge from the blazing beach for a morning. It had a museum of modern art hosting a Picasso exhibition, a natural history museum, churches dripping with history and streets that demanded to be strolled down. My first port of call? The home of Tenerife FC. Dad's weird habits are infecting me this holiday. A huge mural on the side of the stadium paid homage to a former player from the 1980s called Rommel Fernández. I love the fact that every football club has a cult hero. I'm still in love with York City legend Keith Walwyn.

Saturday 10 July

My first funeral visit. At Sarah Bulmer's house. If I overthought how weird life is sometimes my head would explode. The last time we were together I was dressed in my hideous porter's uniform. I was trying to woo her with cheeky banter in a Posthouse bathroom. Now I've got to lay her dad to rest. Surreal. Sarah immediately cut through the tension by reminding me of the excruciating love poems I used to send her. Ouch. She's had a really tough few years. The father of her daughter called off their wedding with three weeks to go. Now she has lost her dad to cancer. I sat in the front room as Sarah and her close family told me about Bob. He was adored.

Tuesday 13 July

As I looked out over the packed crematorium at Bob's funeral I had a moment of clarity. My knees knocked violently. My tongue had turned into sand. I'd become aware of the possibility that I could faint. But then it struck me. The reality and truth of my calling swept over me. I wouldn't capitulate. I would be strong and lead these grieving people. God was with me. This was me now. I took a deep, deliberate breath and I began to speak. The rest is a blur. Bob was mourned with laughter and tears. An extract from The Kinks' song 'Days' was read out. It sounded like the most poignant of prayers. 'Those sacred days you gave me …' I know I'll take countless funerals in my life, but this first one will always be special.

Wednesday 14 July

I had a bizarre conversation with the owner of a sandwich shop this morning. I'd gone in there to read my Bible and drink strong coffee. He took the exchanging of a few pleasantries as an invitation to join me at the table. Clearly he had things to get off his chest. He broke into a rant about the rudeness of his customers. 'I say good morning to them and they just totally ignore me, so I tell them to f*** off out of the shop,' he said, his face going from pink to red to deep purple. He claimed that vicars and teachers were the worst offenders. His wife looked over in despair from behind the counter. I bet she gets both barrels.

As I prepared to leave, he suddenly asked me how I found God. I gave him the short version. His face softened after that. A strange peace invaded the space between us. I was so struck by how much this guy needed the love of God in his life. I made a point of saying 'goodbye' and 'thank you' at terrific volume as I walked out. Just in case he thought about telling me to 'f*** off'.

Anna was in good spirits tonight. She looks big and delicious. We listened to our favourite Shed Seven songs while doing the pots and jumped around the kitchen playing air guitar.

Sunday 18 July

I've sorted out the old *Evening Press* cuttings from my days working with Dennis in the Selby office. Nostalgia swept over me. Dennis knew people better than anyone I've ever met. There weren't many immune to his understated charms. His powers of persuasion were legendary. But he was as kind and pastoral as any priest when dealing with distressed people.

Dennis taught me how to see beyond the relative mundanity of life in Selby and Tadcaster. He could unearth outrage, intrigue and human drama during the quietest news days. It didn't feel like learning the journalistic dark arts but rather an education in connecting with all kinds of people – from striking bin men to mad aristocrats. Of course, leafing through the clippings, I see now that I overegged the pudding at times. I overstepped the mark. But I give thanks for those years. Becoming a reverend will not be so different, I suspect. It's all about people.

Monday 19 July

Anna and I are sat in bed in glorious Whitby discussing possible baby names. It dominates our conversations. If they're boys we'll call them Freddie Romero and Raphael John. One of the girls will be called Heidi Mae. Anna also likes Esther. I can't stop thinking about the possibility of us moving to Hull. I meet Holy Trinity's vicar, Neal, on Thursday. Is this where God is calling us?

Driving to Whitby over the North York Moors is spectacular. Going past the nuclear missile early warning station base at RAF

Fylingdales always reminds me of my press interview with Thom Yorke from Radiohead. He was leading a protest march. We sat on a rock while he raged about the dangers of weapons of mass destruction. I wasn't really listening. All I could think about was that this man made one of my favourite albums, *OK Computer.* I got my picture with him before he set off with his megaphone. Thom doesn't smile much.

Whitby is so wonderfully familiar to us. After a walk, a snooze and a pint we queued for an hour to get a table at the Magpie. We became engrossed in a blazing row a young couple were having behind us. I think she had a point. He does sound like he's been going out with his friends too much and not pulling his weight round the house. I'm glad we queued. These are the best fish and chips in the world.

Tuesday 20 July

Our B&B owner is from Venezuela. She's feisty and eccentric. She called me a 'grumpy git' as she served us our poached eggs this morning. Brilliant.

Thursday 22 July

I instantly liked the Reverend Neal Barnes when I met him at his vicarage today. You couldn't fail to. He is warm, kind, gentle and honest. There's a lovely holiness to him. Neal is also wonderfully uncool. He reeked of Radio 4 and gardening. Almost inevitably, paintings of steam trains adorned his office wall. (What is it with vicars and trains?!) Neal said he'd heard about my work with blokes but admitted to not being much of a 'man's man'. I confessed that I could be irritable, impatient and grumpy to work with. He said he admired that level of honesty and self-awareness. The more we tried to put each other off the more we became bonded. If we worked together, Neal promised to give me the freedom to pioneer new things.

In describing the state of Holy Trinity he did not hang back. It felt like he was warning me against going there. He described it as not so much being in the hospital needing a doctor, but in the morgue needing to be raised to life. It is haemorrhaging cash (losing at least £1,000 a week), congregation numbers have severely declined, there's little going on apart from the usual Sunday services and it has virtually no community engagement.

As Neal talked, my insides began to flutter as I imagined God using me to help breathe new life into it. I said I loved a challenge. He agreed with my belief that church should be a place of prayer and parties. Before long we were plotting together what Holy Trinity needed – discipleship, community involvement and lots of evangelism going on to grow it. This was a significant meeting. I came away feeling uplifted and excited. My instincts tell me that I could work with Neal. But is this what God wants? And can Anna be persuaded that this is what she wants?

Friday 23 July

I met Anna after she finished work to talk about Holy Trinity. I expressed my excitement at the possibility of us going there. She is stressed and worried at the thought of leaving York. Crying and snotting into a tissue, she said: 'I do not want to move, Woody.' It was fairly categorical. I did my best to reassure her that Hull was only an hour away and we'd come back regularly. She has at least agreed to come and look at the house.

I popped into the communications office at Bishopthorpe Palace to catch up on some work I'd done for the Archbishop's Youth Trust charity. When Sentamu saw me, he sang that line from Morning Prayer: 'O Lord, open our lips!' I sang back: 'And our mouth shall proclaim your praise!' He joked that if I don't take the Hull job, he'd give me something *really* hard.

I went to Aunty Lynne's for lunch. She looked gaunt from the chemotherapy but her hair hasn't fallen out, which is a relief. Uncle Ally persuaded me to sign on for Long Marston's second XI cricket team again. Any time spent with them at the moment is a gift.

Saturday 24 July

It was a long day of partying and socializing to celebrate Ian's 40th. I've never seen York races so busy. There was hardly a spare inch of grass. As Ian's friends gathered by the paddock I hit it off with the husband of one of his teaching assistants. Alex is a major in the army and about to embark on a six-month tour in Afghanistan next month. I later asked him to email me his updates and said I'd commit to pray for him while he was away. We danced and sang our hearts out to the *X-Factor* finalists during the post-race entertainment. How embarrassing.

Ian had hired buses to take us to his evening do at the university. Things got very silly. I belted out a spontaneous rap about having a low sperm count. I'm praying it doesn't surface on social media. At 2 a.m. the late stragglers joined arms to sing 'My Way' before getting the bus home.

Sunday 25 July

I felt wretched after last night's frivolities. Some of my behaviour was far from priestly. And yet even in the middle of such a raucous knees up, God was at work. Why am I surprised? Major Alex emailed to thank me for offering to pray when he goes to Afghanistan. Anna is all at sea at the possibility of moving. Everything I do and say is wrong. I'm getting snapped at. A lot. The last thing I want is to force her to move somewhere that will make her so unhappy. She has to feel called to Hull too.

Saturday 31 July

Aunty Lynne's chemotherapy treatment hasn't worked. The lump in her throat has actually got bigger. Jo is understandably angry with God. She asked Mum why he has granted us two miracles but not one for them. It's a fair question. I wish I knew. I know God works in mysterious ways, but sometimes I wish he wouldn't. We want clarity, answers. Aunty Lynne has turned down Mum's offer of prayer. She wants to get through it her own way. It's devastating. I got the chance to spend some time with her at the cricket match against Garforth. Uncle Ally is putting a brave face on, but I noticed such pain in his eyes.

Sunday 1 August

Our visit to Hull to look round Holy Trinity and the curate's house was disastrous. A car crash of tears, blazing rows and tense silences. And that was just on the drive there. Anna aside, everything feels right about moving here. But there is no 'Anna aside'. None of this works without her blessing. Unless she can see her mother from our bathroom window she's openly hostile to moving anywhere – let alone a city that is bottom of most lists it wants to be top of and top of most lists it wants to be bottom of.

As a reporter, I mastered the art of persuading people to do stuff they didn't really want to do. Convincing Anna to do this may be beyond me, though. In the car, the more her face turned to thunder, the more my frustrations became vocalized. Minutes after we pulled up outside the curate's house, one of the neighbours told us that there was a twins' club in the local community centre. Surely that's a positive sign? Surely this generated a flicker of excitement in Anna? Surely it thawed the ice a bit? No. Nothing. Inevitably we descended into a full-scale row outside the property that we will probably never live in now.

We walked in silence to explore Holy Trinity. It's massive – like God's aircraft hangar. The service was just finishing when we rocked up. The congregation was small. There didn't seem to be any non-grey heads among them. The worship was formal and word-heavy. Holy Trinity is 700 years old. I'm not convinced they'd be ready for my kind of change. Outside there was more potential. There's a great square surrounded by pubs and shops. Anna's sulking and sobbing reached biblical proportions on the way home. She kept saying that it would be my decision to move. I didn't cover myself in glory with my reply. Anna says I have a 'forked tongue'. My words too often hit the hurt spot. What are we going to do?

Tuesday 3 August

Anna had her 20-week scan at York Hospital. We have two healthy babies.

Friday 6 August

I'm struggling to sleep. I can't stop thinking about my decision to leave journalism to work for the Church ('from news to pews' as the *Press* lads put it). It feels like utter madness now. The power of spiritual moments like I experienced that day on the A19 to Selby become diminished over time. I often ask myself if it ever really happened. I'm glad I wrote it down. Back then I was sure enough to leave the career I loved, and any semblance of financial security. I can still picture my editor crying with laughter when I told him why I was handing my notice in. Dad was so upset that he refused to come to my leaving do. He missed an epic night at the Tap and Spile.

On these nights of doubt, I try to remember those who were impacted by my calling. Like my old friend Tom. He was in danger of killing himself with vodka. Persuading him to get help and come to church changed everything. Within 18 months he was sober and kneeling before a bishop to be confirmed. He was bathed in an unforgettable serenity that night.

As I write this, Anna has just sworn at me for giving her a light poke. Her pregnancy snores aren't funny any more. It's like trying to sleep next to Bernard Manning with a cold.

Saturday 7 August

Aunty Lynne has had a bad week. In my morning quiet time, I prayed that she'd be completely healed. I tried to muster the faith that God could and would do it. Spiritual healing leaves me racked with doubts and questions. Why does God choose to heal some and not others? I recently witnessed a charismatic church leader praying for someone. He rebuked the illness in the name of Jesus like it was some kind of demon. Like it was somehow the fault of the afflicted. I struggle with the theology and morality of that approach. It's a potential minefield. I'm struggling with the theology of many things right now. My summer placements have left me with far more questions than answers. Maybe that's the point?

I played cricket for Long Marston today. As we waited to bat, grizzled, cynical old Keith bombarded me with questions about prayer and priests. He asked if I was able to administer the last rites. 'Thorner's bowlers aren't that quick, Keith!' I joked. Keith is typical of many people. He has no real interest in making a spiritual commitment but wants to know if he'll be OK when he eventually stops breathing. It dawned on me, when he eventually went out to the middle, that running between those wickets on a diet of fried breakfasts, cigars and single malts it might happen sooner than he thinks. As it turned out he was out third ball. He disappeared into the changing room in a puff of profanity and cigar smoke.

I arrived home to be greeted by a delicious seafood risotto and bottle of red. I love that Anna would think of doing that.

We watched *Changing Lanes*. It's the third film I've seen recently about morally suspect lawyers. It made me think about my own sense of morality while working as a reporter at the *Evening Press*. There were times when I crossed the line. Our budget didn't stretch to phone hacking. But I too often manipulated people with charismatic word-smithery into telling me things that they didn't really want to. And then posing for a picture.

Sunday 8 August

I'm back in North Wales to be a tent leader at Pathfinder Camp for the first time in ten years. So much of my teenage years and early twenties were defined by this holiday. The drive over the hill into Criccieth to be greeted by the rugged coastline and castle ruins is still jaw-dropping. Nothing seems to have changed. Driving onto the field, camp even had the same smell. Once all the leaders had arrived, I was asked to say a few words about why I'd come back after so long. I shared that I wanted to remind myself why I was a Christian. This was the place where the gospel first came alive to me. Training at vicar factory has a tendency to knock some of the joy and wonder of it out of you. Many of my heroes and role models were leaders here, I said. Our younger generation now needed heroes more than ever. I must have sounded like a right old fart!

We later went for a pint to the Bryn Hir Arms. As we pulled up outside, a fight was breaking out between a gang of lads. In the confusion, one of them thought I was involved. He pointed to his bloodied friend and shouted at me: 'Your mate glassed him in the face!' I quickly explained that we were leaders on a Christian camp who'd come for a quiet drink. That told him.

Tuesday 10 August

I'd forgotten how exhausting camp is. It dawned on me that I'd been running about for four hours – and it was only 9.30 a.m. There are some really edgy, broken kids here. One lad told me that his dad wanted nothing to do with him. His home life sounded grim. These ten days will hopefully show him that the world can be full of goodness and hope. The lads in my tent are really opening up before lights out. We go from discussing the eternal mysteries of faith and the universe to which girls on camp are in their top five (in reverse order).

Thursday 12 August

After morning games, Anna and I walked into Criccieth for another summit about moving to Hull. Initially, she was angry and tearful but then – to my surprise – began to talk more reasonably and realistically. Deep down, I'm pretty sure she wants this adventure but the thought of having the twins and not being within hugging distance of her mum hurts her deeply. After an intense, difficult discussion, Anna said she had two conditions to moving. The first is that we come back to York after three years. The second is that I'll take her back to York whenever she feels homesick or wants to see her mum. I couldn't agree to them. We can't put conditions on a divine calling.

Saturday 14 August

The whole camp went to see Porthmadog FC play Cefn Druids this afternoon. It was like Christmas for the lady running the club shop. We cleared out the place, gobbling up Porthmadog hats, scarves and hoodies. We crowded in behind the away goal, trebling the attendance.

A holy moment passed between us as a tent tonight. We laid on our backs in an open bit of the field to gaze up at the stars. We talked about the possibility of other worlds, the vastness of the universe and the majesty of God's creation. And girls. They won't shut up about girls. Before turning in, we were treated to the most spectacular shooting star. It flashed and blazed above us. I hope it was a moment these lads will always remember. My heart is bursting with joy at serving God here.

Sunday 15 August

Being so close to nature and living so simply at camp is doing special things to me. Ryan dragged me up at 6 a.m. for a run and swim in the sea. The sun was coming up over the mountains in the distance. We floated on our backs in the water and talked about deep things. It was a moment to feel utterly privileged to be alive. God has become real again. Close. Not just someone we discuss in a seminar.

Monday 16 August

I took a mini-bus full of campers seal-watching to Nefyn. I stupidly promised that they would *definitely* see some. The campers had reached a fever pitch of excitement by the time we got to the vantage point. Unfortunately, the sea was entirely empty of seals. The look of disappointment on their young faces was awful. We waited and waited. Nothing. I was just about to make the call to head back when, in a moment of pure magic, a seal's head suddenly popped out of the water. And then another one! It was like a scene from a film. I whooped and hollered and danced around on the rocks as the kids' cameras clicked into action. We ended the trip with ice cream and cans of Dr Pepper.

Our tent discussion was a lively one after evening meeting tonight. One of the lads wants to pursue a career in the Army. He asked if, in God's eyes, it was wrong for soldiers to kill. I prefer it when they ask me about girls.

Tuesday 17 August

We sneaked our tent lads off the campsite for an adventure after lights out. We all dressed in black and crawled out on our stomachs to evade the patrols. We ran down to the beach with bags of snacks and treats. It was like something from an Enid Blyton novel, only with rough northern teenagers who swear and smoke. We laughed in the face of health and safety, insurance, risk assessments and the actual camp rules. The boys needed this. We sat on the end of the pier eating Hula Hoops and Twiglets, throwing stones into the sea and talking rubbish. They shared their camp highlights and their hopes and fears about going home. I gave each of them a stone to keep somewhere as a reminder that no matter how hard life gets, God was with them always. Frankly, I think they were expecting something a bit more exciting than a stone.

As we sat under the Criccieth moonlight it dawned on me that these boys had helped to reignite my faith and reaffirm my priestly calling. I gave thanks to God for them. We got back to camp undetected. And no one died. Result.

Saturday 21 August

Birthdays are not for me any more. Turning 35 today is a terrible thing. I've got too much to do and see and experience, but time's running out! The flecks of grey in my hair have become whole strands. The creases around my eyes are as deep as wood carvings. And I now sit down when I wee. When did that happen? Yet I feel that Red Bull must be permanently coursing through my veins. My mind is whirring and bubbling constantly with a drive and an urge for new adventures.

Anna cooked me poached eggs to absolute perfection. My birthday gifts included cinema tickets and wine gums. Onwards.

Monday 23 August

Anna has officially agreed to move to Hull. It was dependent on me agreeing to three non-negotiable conditions. She wrote them down on a piece of paper that I reluctantly had to sign. Not in blood, thank goodness. If it gives Anna some peace then so be it. I'm so proud of her. The conditions are:

1. Don't put any pressure on me to leave my job in York.
2. Make every effort to move back to York after 3–4 years if that is what I want.
3. Drive me back to York if I really need you to.

There's a common theme here! The main thing is that the move is on. Excitement is stirring within me. The winds of change – revolution even – are coming to Holy Trinity. I can feel it.

I dropped into Lee's shop for a pork pie to tell him about Hull. We're getting giddy about our big rugby league Challenge Cup weekend. His mum has been out for a few dates. Lee isn't taking it well. I know how he feels. But we've got to let our mums get on with living. It's interesting how they mother us for years and then as we grow older and life gets messy we try to father them.

Tuesday 24 August

I attended Keith's dad's funeral at York crematorium. It was a humanist ceremony but I still found it an intensely spiritual affair. God was in that room whether the humanists liked it or not. Keith wrote a long eulogy about his dad. He talked about them going to see *The Empire Strikes Back* and playing football and cricket in the fields behind their house. I was inspired to call my dad later on and suggest we resume our European tour. We're thinking Belgium or Poland. You only get one dad.

Sunday 29 August

Lee built up our Challenge Cup weekend so much that it could never live up to it. There were great moments of bonding and fun but we largely spoilt it with our bickering and desire to be right. It reached fever pitch at the Chandos. We tried to dissect why we'd reached such a low ebb in our friendship this weekend. Lee thinks I have a huge ego and that life always has to revolve around me. I responded that he was too often mean, negative and critical of friends' bodies and clothes as a way of masking his own insecurities. The honesty was good. With the air cleared, we bought cans of Fosters and laughed all the way home on the train. Secretly, though, I suspect both of us are wounded by our harsh analysis of each other. I know I am.

Monday 30 August

Anna too often gets the dregs of me. Things were a bit strained as we ate our sausage casserole tonight. Watching *Jerry Maguire* saved the day. We drew closer as the love grew between Tom Cruise and Renée Zellweger on screen. 'You had me at hello' is the greatest line in rom-com.

Tuesday 31 August

I met my old friend Simon in Costa to unpack my recent church placement. We got onto the problem of suffering, the delights of Rowan Williams, homosexuality, speaking in tongues and indie rock. Simon is that rare combination of someone who is interesting and interested.

As a relatively new Christian, he's struggling with his church's stance on homosexuality. His girlfriend stormed out of one of the services after the preacher claimed that single-parent families were 'generating' more gay people because of absent fathers. The pastor went on to argue that you could always tell when a society is on the verge of moral collapse because homosexuals are a dominant force. I told Simon that some churches become so consumed by the gay issue that they neglect the stuff Jesus actually preached about – serving, loving, caring, accepting and not judging others. It seems to me that we've got our work cut out with that lot before falling out over something that Jesus never actually mentioned. Jesus never discriminated. Neither should we.

Thursday 2 September

Dad was on electric form when I met him in Nero's. He's passionate about our big move to Hull. He drew me a rough map of the city on a napkin. Annoying amounts of geographical knowledge inhabit this man's brain. An hour with Dad and I'm excited at the prospect of living there. He's a tonic to those who've responded to our news with thinly veiled disbelief and derision. 'What yer moving there fer? It's a right s***hole!' has been a typical response. It's so uninformed and unhelpful.

Dad has agreed to give me a tour in a few weeks. He knows the area around Holy Trinity well from his press days. Our conversation then turned to the genius of Alex Higgins. Dad had seen a documentary about him last night that made him cry. Just hearing about it made me cry. I watched it when I got home. I cried again. What is wrong with me?

Friday 3 September

I called up Ronnie at his care home. He's sounding very frail. He spurned my offer to visit him. He said he was too old, confused and suffering from narcolepsy. He then went into his usual rant about the abuses in the Catholic Church. I suggested he might try to differentiate between the evil that men do and the love of God. He accused me of treating him like a teenager. That call went well then.

Tuesday 7 September

I keep thinking about Lee's comments during the Challenge Cup weekend in London. They've hurt and challenged me. He claimed our friends sometimes avoid me because I talk and boast about myself too much. Is it hurting because it's the truth? Certainly, I don't know anyone who falls out with their mates as much as me. There's always some ongoing conflict or issue with one of them. It's a constant carousel of pushing them away and pulling them close. I blame my parents.

Wednesday 8 September

Major Alex has emailed me from his base in Afghanistan. He thanked me for the comfort cross I sent and the prayers I'm praying. He's missing his family.

Thursday 9 September

I settled myself into a huge comfy chair in Starbucks to people-watch over a main shopping street in Harrogate. There was a huge kerfuffle outside the Marks and Spencer opposite after a power cut forced it to close. A nervous-looking junior manager in a creased shirt had the difficult job of informing customers. They weren't happy. It got me thinking about church and how people would react if that was forced to close on Sunday. Would folk be as bothered? Sadly, probably not. Shops seem to be the modern places of worship now. The M&S counter is the new altar.

I texted Lee to draw a line under our recent conflicts. It said: 'Lee, you said some things that really hurt me and I know I did to you. But you are my best friend and I love you so we need to move on. I'm sorry. Let's move on. OK?' Saying sorry always feels good. Lee's reply was short, to the point and tinged with an obvious embarrassment to be even having this kind of exchange with another male. 'OK, boss', he wrote.

Saturday 11 September

I stumbled across an uncomfortable quote from Stephen Fry today. It said that if God existed and if the Church of England was any part of his plan for the world, why would he choose such 'dorks' to be priests? He has a point. What Fry doesn't grasp is that God is in the business of making treasure out of jars of clay. And dorky priests.

It has been one of those days when I'm racked with doubts about faith and God. How did Christ's message get so shockingly twisted? Flicking through the Christian satellite TV channels at Amy and Keith's house didn't help. Too many of the presenters were reassuring viewers that they could secure miracles for the right price. One horribly tanned preacher was asking viewers to send him exactly 58 dollars. That was the amount he needed to 'release the blessing'. This is the new heresy.

We went to a posh 70th birthday party tonight. I borrowed a tuxedo and spent far too long in front of the mirror recreating the opening credits scene from the James Bond movies when he walks and turns to shoot at the camera. Anna looked delicious and pregnant in a little black dress. It cried out for a speed boat for us to climb into. The No. 5 bus to New Earswick didn't quite do it.

Monday 13 September

Dad is the most gifted enthusiast. In the space of six hours, he made moving to Hull feel like the only viable option in life. He gave me a tour of the atmospheric cobbled streets in the Old Town that are part of my parish. Dad pointed out places and buildings of interest. He waxed lyrical about the 'Victorian façades' and 'marvellous little boozers'. We visited Holy Trinity and our new house, before taking stock at the Olde White Harte. The upstairs room was where the decision that sparked the English Civil War was taken. Allegedly.

Dad smashed his head against the low-hanging glass rack above the bar. He swore loudly and hilariously. The landlord thought he was insane. He's very familiar with these pubs from his press days. Come to think of it, he's familiar with many pubs from his press days. It wasn't a day's work if the hacks back then hadn't supped six pints over lunchtime. I remember the smell of beer and fags on him when he got home to us in Murray Street. Ironically, that seemed to be the only place Dad wasn't very enthusiastic about.

Tuesday 14 September

Mum booked me in at the orthodontist this morning. She's become an evangelist for the place after getting a brace fitted to straighten her teeth. The specialist guessed that I still sucked my thumb. How embarrassing. He shared his best technique to stop – wearing a sock on my hand when I go to bed. I expected a more scientific remedy, to be honest.

I've discovered a wonderful piece of music on Classic FM called 'O Magnum Mysterium' by a composer called Morten Lauridsen. As Simon Bates told his listeners: 'It's like the entrance music to heaven.' Cheese. Anna is at 26 weeks today.

Reading Genesis continues to surprise and shock. Today's chapter was about a bloke who was having sex with his brother's wife. He 'spilt his seed on the ground' after pulling out at the crucial moment so as not to get her pregnant. God struck him down. Ouch.

My old church buddy Josh came round for a brew this afternoon. He always illuminates my day. We flew a kite in West Bank Park. The string kept getting snagged in the trees so we sneaked onto the bowling green where there was more room. The park keeper busted us. He was very unhappy. It was like being transported back to 1987 when I'd be reprimanded for various misdemeanours with my smoking buddies. Trainee vicars should not still be getting thrown out of parks.

Wednesday 15 September

For the first time in over 20 years I didn't suck my thumb in bed last night. I wore a plaster in case I got tempted. The buck teeth stop here.

I visited Darren in Wealstun Prison near Wetherby this morning. He's been inside for just over a year now and gets out in ten weeks. It worries me that he's already making plans to go back on the booze. It's what got him in there in the first place. 'My mam says it's the spirits what do me in,' Darren told me. 'I'll be OK with beer.' Will he ever learn? We embraced at the end in the middle of that grim visiting room. Screaming children had to be peeled off their dads. I prayed that God would protect Darren during his remaining stint.

Thursday 16 September

I nearly died tonight. Time does stand still. You do have a real clarity of thought in those milliseconds. I'd been driving back from Neal's licensing service at Holy Trinity. He's now officially the vicar there – and my boss from July. It was dark and the roads past South Cave were deceiving. I was going too fast for one particularly tight corner. A car was coming the other way. I slammed all on, the wheels locked and I skidded towards the oncoming car. It's at that point the world slowed right down and my jeans nearly went from blue to brown. I don't think it's too dramatic to say that my life hung in the balance in that moment. As it happened I frantically worked the steering wheel and ended up careering into a hedge. There's no relief like escaping death. I pulled into a layby to call Anna. I needed to hear her voice. I'm determined not to die before I hold our two babies. There's nothing like a near-death experience to help you appreciate life.

Neal's big night at Holy Trinity was well attended. The church was freezing. I get the impression this place needs warming up in

122

every sense. Starting with the choir. Talk about worshipping the Lord with joy and gladness. They looked like they were having a very bad year.

The Bishop of Hull was on good form. I liked the way he articulated the fact that radical change happens at Holy Trinity or it dies. He thanked the priests who'd gone before and the church stalwarts for keeping it going. Then came the challenge. Richard warned that there was a danger that people could look at a huge church building like this being empty as a sign that God came to earth and then left it. It's basically three years away from being mothballed. To conclude the service, Richard prayed these powerful words over Neal: 'Keep your eyes fixed on Jesus who was wounded for our sins, that you may bear in your life and ministry the love and joy and peace which are the marks of Jesus in his disciples.' Bishop Richard told me afterwards that a formal letter is being sent to offer me the curacy place at Holy Trinity. I'm just happy to be alive to receive it.

Monday 20 September

I overdosed on Bob Dylan today. It's a surefire sign that I'm feeling melancholy – or have a 'face like a slapped a***', as Anna so eloquently put it. She got the brunt of it. Deep down I'm scared about leaving her to go back to Durham. We had some grumpy exchanges in Tesco. She went to bed hours ago. I'm back at Cranmer in ten days. We have two babies on the way. Tomorrow, I need to fast, pray, read and ponder my way out of these black clouds. And no more Bob Dylan.

Tuesday 21 September

I slept in the spare room last night. Anna's snoring was unbearable and I needed to be alone. I've spent the day fasting and retreating from the world. I'm devouring an essential book for all would-be priests: David Bosch's masterful *Transforming Mission*. There's not a lot of gags in it, but it's so full of truth, outstanding theology and helpful biblical insights. His words get into your head, and flow down to your heart. Bosch makes you want to actually get out of the library and onto the street. It's what highlighter pens were made for. Bosch says that 'Christians find their true identity when they are involved in mission, in communicating to others a new way of life, a new interpretation of reality and of God, and in committing themselves to the liberation and salvation of others.' And I need to remember this insight when I start in Hull: 'Mission never takes place in self-confidence but in the knowledge of our own weakness, at a point of crisis where danger and opportunity come together.' Bosch reminded me today that nothing has changed. St Paul was the first pioneer minister. Bosch writes: 'Paul's ministry thus unfolds in a creative tension between loyalty to the first apostles and their message on the one hand and an overpowering awareness of the uniqueness of his own calling and commission on the other.' In other words, Paul had to be brave and bring the change. I must be too.

I hugely benefited from some stillness before God today. I never seem to learn that we can't expect to hear from him if we don't actually make time to listen. The only way he seems to speak to me is in the silence.

Anna and I watched *The Back-up Plan* tonight. It's about Jennifer Lopez getting a sperm donor and giving birth to twins. It was cheese on toast but made Anna laugh. That made me happy.

Thursday 23 September

Bosch gave me a whistle-stop tour through hundreds of years of church history today. Fascinating. In the Enlightenment period, people were deceived into thinking that they didn't need God any more. They began to believe that science, reason and human progress could answer all their questions and make their lives complete. They were wrong.

I went from the intellectual, theological denseness of Bosch to the earthiness of Acomb Working Men's Club. It was no less fascinating. Anna's brother was in there, playing fives and threes with an old guy called Ernie. I'd done press stories on Ernie's son who is a well-known Elvis impersonator. Ernie cleans drains for a living. He was fascinated by my calling to the priesthood. We got onto the subject of monks. He shared a brilliant story about working at Ampleforth Abbey. He'd asked one of the brothers to show him where to find the hot water supply. Ernie was escorted down to the cellar where he noticed a huge barrel of cider. It was 10 a.m. Ernie and the monk re-emerged at 1.30 p.m. totally plastered. 'That was one of the best sessions I ever had!' he cackled.

Sunday 26 September

All day I chewed over this quote from Allan Bloom's *The Closing of the American Mind*:

> *individuals can no longer take themselves seriously and that, in spite of the fact that they now have the liberty to believe and do as they like, many do not believe in anything any more, and all spend their lives in frenzied work and frenzied play so as not to face the fact, not to look into the abyss.*

I reject this. Most people still have an innate desire to believe in something. That inner spiritual thirst is there somewhere. Surely? When people are brave enough, compelled enough, to slow the frenzy of work and play and stop gorging on the fleeting pleasures of shopping, sex, footy, lager and tacky TV, the bigger questions of life, a deeper truth, will emerge. Whenever I come out in a cold sweat, traumatized at the potential that God doesn't exist, that I'm talking to myself in prayer, my thoughts turn to Jesus. He draws me back to belief. He restores my hope. He pulls me from the abyss.

Admittedly, I had a night off the bigger questions of life. I indulged in rubbish telly, a few cans of lager and an early night with Anna.

Wednesday 29 September

I'm getting jittery about going back to college. Essays will soon be coming out of my ears. It will take huge amounts of self-discipline to juggle the work, and then come back to York at weekends to be a dad to two screaming babies. One of them keeps having a disco in Anna's womb. Putting my ear to her tummy is now my new favourite thing to do in the entire world. We went out for a meal after getting more Tesco vouchers. On the way out we pulled each other close in the hallway and petted heavily.

Thursday 30 September

It was great to see all the boys at Cranmer again. I'm living in college this year next door to Paul Bromley. Things should be easier and much more fun. I won't miss Dan's moody introspection or Phil's shower pubes. After an all-age welcome-back service I met Harry Sawyer who I'll be doing a pioneer placement with. He's a big guy with one of those Middle Eastern beards that doesn't cover the area above his lip. David reassured me – between mouthfuls of quiche – that my family had to come first and I could take whatever time I needed. What a stunning man.

One of the new intake is only nineteen. Nineteen! What's he doing?! I've been assigned to be his 'college buddy' to ensure he settles in. He's very bouncy and smiles for extended periods. I took him to the Elm Tree and the Colpitts to get properly acquainted. I'm not great mentor material. My track record is terrible.

If all goes to plan I'll be a reverend in about nine months. And a dad in less than three. Ouch.

Tuesday 5 October

I felt completely out of my depth in our first Old Testament lecture. We're looking at the wisdom literature contained in books like the Psalms, Proverbs and Ecclesiastes. There were a lot of words being used like 'flux' and 'relativism'. Aidan talked a *lot*. At least 90 per cent of it was absolute garbage. Things didn't get any easier in our systematics seminar. I'm determined to not just get my head round this stuff but find a way to apply it to real life. Systematics seems to boil down to one of two conclusions:

1. The answer is always Jesus.
2. It's all a mystery.

I just need to find some colourful and creative ways of saying that in my essays. We headed to the Colpitts after college Communion. It was hard work maintaining polite conversation with some of our new intake. Hopefully they'll learn to put down those Bible commentaries for the night and engage in some pub banter.

Wednesday 6 October

It doesn't take a psychologist to realize that Anna is trying to prepare me for fatherhood. She has sent me an article about having twins from a male perspective. The guy articulated the enormity of the sacrifice: 'What I couldn't handle, and what put me totally over the edge, was finding out that I had to arrange my entire schedule around the boys. I initially thought that I'd be able to force them onto my schedule, but that just didn't work.' Anna knows me so well. Too well. Her card included this Mother Teresa quote: 'I know God will not give me anything I can't handle. I just wish he didn't trust me so much.' We can do this. I can do this.

Harry and I have embarked on our pioneer placement adventure. Our brief is to familiarize ourselves with the Gilesgate and Sherburn Road estate area of Durham. We will meet the people, listen to God, and make connections with the local churches before presenting a report on our findings. The only thing we can't do is start anything new. That won't be easy for an impatient, restless sod like me. Stuart has called our placement a process of 'deep listening'. Harry and I walked the patch. We bumped into two officers from the community policing team who were really helpful. They said the estate used to be notorious. A virtual no-go area for the emergency services. This will be a good place to learn.

Thursday 7 October

Our New Testament lecturer is a brilliant man but a spiky character. And that's being polite. When one of our class offered a comment that he didn't agree with, he snapped back: 'You are wrong!' I'm hanging onto his every word. It's New Testament gold.

An American priest from Alabama is teaching us Anglicanism. He answers to 'Father'. He began by explaining that our history was one of intense infighting between the three main wings of the Church of England – evangelical, liberal and catholic. Over the years there has been constant tension between them. To be an Anglican is to exist within this tension. It's a weakness and a strength. Former Archbishop Michael Ramsey said that 'Its credentials are its incompleteness with the tension and travail of its soul. It is clumsy and untidy, it baffles neatness and logic.' This describes where I am right now. I am a theological and liturgical magpie. A bit of this. A bit of that. Whatever works.

A St John's College music student called Zach has a room opposite Paul and me on B Floor. We'll have some fun with this guy. I love that the undergrads are mixed in with the trainee revs.

We have a lot to learn from each other. Zach joined us for Compline in the chapel tonight. I asked him later if he thought we were in tune. 'Not really,' he replied.

Friday 8 October

It was interesting to note in our first seminar on leadership that charisma seems to be frowned upon. One quote was read out that said: 'Charisma becomes the undoing of leaders. It makes them inflexible, convinced of their infallibility, unable to change.' Surely it depends on how you define charisma? The Church of England has been churning out too many leaders with a severe lack of it for generations and look at the state we're in. I long to see more vicars with a deep commitment to Christ who'll anger, frustrate, inspire, and make us laugh and cry. We seem scared to death of leaders with a personality.

Generally speaking – many priests in the Church of England seem to be prayerful, introverted, academic and safe. They relate to a certain type of person at a certain type of church. And that's fine. All I'm saying is let's seek to redress the imbalance a bit. Encouraging people into Christian leadership who have an infectious, living faith, and can relate Jesus to the ordinary working man and woman, should now be high priority. Surely? We've ordained generations of clergy who effortlessly talk the language of Radio 4. Let's now ordain a few who talk the language of *Coronation Street*. I'm glad that's off my chest!

Joel Wood has become my spiritual muse. I'm a sponge for his passion, wisdom and thirst for Christ. We got deep over a beer in the Shakespeare tonight. He's had a call from a top screenwriter he knows from his writing days. She wants his help on developing a new TV detective series. Joel said it feels like a beautiful woman catching his eye in the street and tempting him. A few years ago he'd have done anything to talk to her. Now he's worried that it will take his focus away from being a priest. This is a leader I'd follow.

Saturday 9 October

Anna has come to Cranmer for the night. She makes things nice. She's a nester. My college room now feels like a home. She's decked it out in lamps and candles and quality drapery. Our babies are sucking Anna dry of nutrients. Her gums are swollen and bloodied. Her chin is covered in spots. But my heart still pounds with an intense love for her.

We went for a meal to Jason and Ruth's house tonight. Jason says they have the 'spiritual gift of hospitality'. Who says that? He has a point, though. The dining table was more appropriate for a state visit. I felt like the Chilean ambassador taking my seat. It was adorned with candles in ornate silver holders. Rolled napkins were laid out at exact angles. Best of all, our place names were written out in flowery calligraphy. I tried really hard to be civilized and not dominate the conversation. Results were mixed once the wine flowed. I have the spiritual gift of talking crap.

Wednesday 13 October

Anna called me in a state of tearful panic tonight. She'd fallen downstairs. Thank the Lord she slid down on her back. The babies seem fine. Anna checked their heartbeats to be sure. It was a scare we don't need right now. The whole thing feels precarious again just when I was beginning to relax.

My 'college buddy' says he is struggling to cope with the fawning attention of the female undergrads. I can't imagine what it must be like training here as a 19-year-old. The poor guy must be bouncing off the walls. He doesn't seem too distressed by all the attention, mind you.

Thursday 14 October

I dragged myself up at 6.30 a.m. to run with Rhys Thomas. We beat our personal best by one minute. Durham's hills are brutal.

I've received another email from Major Alex in response to the package I sent him. He's doing well but missing his family. Eleven weeks is a long time when you're stuck in a desert wasteland surrounded by local people who want to kill you. He sent me some cool pictures of him posing in a Blackhawk helicopter.

Father Mark's seminars continue to fascinate me. Our class is a lovely cross section of the different Anglican traditions we're learning about. Mark told us that, contrary to popular belief, there were actually fewer people going to church in the seventeenth century than there are now. Anglicanism was on the verge of extinction until the evangelistic preaching ministry of three men changed everything – John and Charles Wesley and George Whitefield. We need a new generation of Wesleys and Whitefields to get busy. Starting with me.

Friday 15 October

Our pioneer ministry seminar was a tasty one. I argued that as a Church we had become 'dangerously irrelevant' to huge swathes of society and urgently needed to re-engage. Aidan and I joked about the potential of 'Matt Woodcock Ministries'. We even came up with a theme tune for the inevitable advert on God TV.

There doesn't seem to be a chapter of the Bible that isn't disputed or questioned in some way in our Cranmer seminars. There's a lot of chin-stroking, brow-furrowing and 'mmm'-ing. It wearies me. We were presented with a hermeneutical analysis on Jesus' central claim of being 'the way, the truth and the life'. Our lecturer claimed it may not be saying what we think it is. For instance, it doesn't rule out the potential that there are other gods. The annoying thing is that this was just left there …

hanging. They leave us standing on theological sand the whole time. We also got onto the thorny issue of universalism (the idea that everyone gets to be with God in heaven in the end, such is the extent of his love and mercy). Our lecturer admitted to not knowing what to make of it but conceded that we'd all love it to be true. Can we be 'certain' about anything written in the New Testament? It would be helpful to know. I know the point of theological training is for me to test and stretch the boundaries of what I know and believe. It would be nice if I didn't actually lose my faith in the process, though.

Sunday 17 October

Harry and I were interviewed at a Methodist church in our placement patch today. I could tell the minister instantly regretted giving me the microphone. I shared how lovely it was to be in a nice warm building with comfy chairs instead of cold, hard pews. 'My bottom thanks you!' I shouted. Cue a wave of embarrassed silence broken by nervous coughs. Cringe.

Monday 18 October

Terrible start to the day. I looked at my alarm clock and saw 6.30 a.m. I showered and liberally applied my Lynx Africa. Glancing at the clock again, I noticed it was actually 3.30 a.m. No! I put a towel over my pillowcase and tried to get back to sleep. I later feigned illness to skip discipleship group. My impression of a chesty cough is getting rather good. I just couldn't face it. I needed to crack on with my essay.

I'm trying to hide from my neighbour Zach. He's a lovely guy but I need more alone time. He keeps sticking rude messages on my door with Post-it notes and coming round to share silly banter. It's like being in one of those frat houses. If I'm not careful Zach will start letting cattle loose down the corridors. Paul says I suffer from IFS (Instant Friend Syndrome). I'm the worst kind of extravert. I only want to be one when I'm in the mood. Then I'm the most extreme type of one. At all other times I need to be quiet and alone. People struggle with the extremity of that transition. I'm a walking Nirvana song – quiet-loud, quiet-loud. It's exhausting.

I ran, observed and prayed the seven miles round our placement patch this afternoon. The big superstores are the new community gathering places. I'm arranging a meeting with the manager of the local Tesco. They could have some useful insights. I'm seeing the area at the moment but not feeling it. I can't hear its heartbeat yet.

Wednesday 20 October

We have a new niece! Elsie Graham came into the world at about 7 a.m. today. Sarah cut the cord. Rob – sensibly – stayed head end. I hope and pray that our babies come out just as smoothly.

Thursday 21 October

Paul Bromley's snoring is becoming a big issue. It was relentless through the night, no matter how much I banged on the wall. He doesn't sound human.

It's great to be with the Morning Glory guys again. We prayed for Sanjay and his marriage. He shared that Menaka had accidentally set part of herself on fire this week. Aidan told us that Claire's health is only at 30 per cent. The drugs aren't working. He fears that she is finally succumbing to the cystic fibrosis. Jason is worried that his depression will resurface as the dark nights close in. So there was a lot to keep God busy with. But we did remember to thank him too. We acknowledged the answers to prayer within the group. I floated out of there on a spiritual high.

Monday 25 October

A new student has joined the community on placement from Lesotho. He's a serious young man called Thapelo. His home life is as primitive as it gets. He goes everywhere by donkey. Being at Cranmer will be a major culture shock.

Anna is 32 weeks pregnant.

Tuesday 26 October

Walter Brueggemann's writing on the Psalms is about the first thing I've understood in Old Testament this term. He says the Psalms present the reader with a three-fold spiritual journey of 'orientation, desolation and reorientation'. This book doesn't flinch from all aspects of the human condition – the good, the bad and the ugly. I don't think God minds us railing at him in anger or desperation. He just hates it when we ignore him. Faith only works in relationship.

Friday 29 October

I felt so invigorated and alive after a 6.30 a.m. run with Joel and Rhys. I burst into the college breakfast room and shouted: 'It's Friday!!' Not everyone shared my morning exuberance.

Our leadership seminar got tasty. The general consensus was that not all ordained people are called to 'lead'. What absolute nonsense! I argued that when we are plonked into a church setting someone has to be its driving force. Our dog collars are a clue as to who that might be. The congregation are relying on us to lead them. Who else is going to do it? It's our calling.

Harry found the idea of vision and long-term planning at odds with the leading and prompting of the Holy Spirit. He would. I hit back that without a flexible strategy for growth, churches are like ships without a rudder. Fatima annoyed me by suggesting that churches should learn how to 'fail well'. She said there were great examples of that being modelled around the UK. Fail well? I said the Church had been failing really well for the last 50 years. Failure is not our issue. Surely it's now time to concentrate on succeeding? On flourishing. On bringing new life and growth and hope to the poor, lost and lonely. That would be lovely. I'm up to here with the Church of England 'failing well'.

Saturday 30 October

I'm disgusted with myself. I overdid it last night to the point where Anna had to virtually carry me home. I had no intention of getting into that state but the wine kept coming as quick as the laughs. I didn't think I was going to live until 2 p.m. today.

Anna and I have been married six years today. What a rollercoaster. We remembered Robin's sermon at our wedding service. He said – metaphorically speaking – that we had a choice in our marriage over whether we choose water or wine. Safety or adventure. Getting by or going for it. I hope we've chosen wine. And not just the kind I did last night. Anna loved my card depicting the spot where I proposed to her on Holy Island.

I've cancelled Ollie's visit to Durham on Thursday. I could just imagine us dancing in Klutes nightclub and the phone going off in my pocket. 'It's Anna – my waters have broken. Get here quickly!' I'm still trying to get my head round the fact that our house will soon echo to the sound of two screaming babies.

Anna and I went to Hotel du Vin for our anniversary meal. They had a deal on. Unfortunately, like a lot of these upmarket places, the staff were *very* attentive. I hate it when waiters are trained to make pally conversation with diners in the hope that they will buy more stuff. They seem to have a list of stock questions like 'How was your day?', spoken in an infuriatingly breezy, rehearsed way. Or am I just being cynical? We were asked if we wanted wine at least four times. In the end I replied – a bit too tersely: 'If you'd have seen me last night you would not be asking that question.' Our waitress saw the funny side. It was lovely to tell Anna that I loved her in the candlelight. It might be greedy, but I hope we get another 60 years together.

Monday 1 November

Being on the verge of fatherhood is doing funny things to me. I'm plagued with vivid dreams. Last night I found myself in a town being invaded by grotesque pirates. It was chaos as people tried to get away from them. I was frantically looking for my two children – a girl and a boy. It may only have been a dream, but the sense of paternal love flowing through me when I found and held them was so intense. I woke up in tears. Is this what being a dad is like? For the first time ever, I'm longing to be one. I think I can do it.

Poor Anna is struggling under the weight of carrying our babies. She can't get comfortable in any position. She's breathing for three now. Between Paul's man-snores at college and Anna's industrial wheezing at home, attempting to sleep is pointless.

Tuesday 2 November

I'm enjoying the banter with my college neighbour Zach. Running into his bedroom with my shades on to do Stevie Wonder impressions on his Casio keyboard just never stops being funny.

Wednesday 3 November

A lady called Sally Jenkins has taught me more about love, hope, perseverance and the human spirit than 100 sermons ever could. Harry and I met her at the Sherburn Road estate community centre. Sally wouldn't class herself as a card-carrying Christian but she certainly does a great impression of one. When she started working at the centre 20 years ago, Sally told us the estate was a deprived, wild and lawless place. There were 17 burglaries a day along with shootings and arsons. The opening of a huge Tesco nearby resurrected the estate, bringing investment and jobs. Signs of its troubled past are still visible on every street corner in the form of huge CCTV cameras mounted in cages. They look like a Banksy art installation.

Sally is worth five CCTV cameras. She's seen countless 'feral youths' transform their behaviour through consistent love and care. I realized that the community centre does the work the local church should be doing. It's threatened with closure if more grants can't be found before March. It would be catastrophic for the area. I offered to write Sally a press release to highlight their plight. I'll also drum up some letters of support from the college top brass. We're determined to help. I told Sally that we'd pray for the money to come in too. Learning from people like Sally is what our time here is all about. It's what life is about. Christ is at work in her and she doesn't even know it.

Friday 5 November

We were treated to a wonderful guest lecture by a Muslim academic today. It made me embarrassingly aware of my ignorance about the Islamic faith. He said that contrary to media inaccuracies his faith was rooted in the pursuit of peace. His natural wide-eyed wonder about Islam was rather beautiful. We're so often embarrassed or apologetic about our Christian belief.

Saturday 6 November

Reading newspapers rarely makes me feel better about the world. Going through the Bible is not dissimilar at the moment. In my chapter of Exodus this morning it detailed a list of holy laws the Jews had to adhere to before entering the Promised Land. The Law of Moses set out that men should be stoned to death if they committed certain offences. I need some help relating to the God of the Old Testament. He just doesn't seem the same as Jesus Christ.

Sunday 7 November

A heavy day of study. I spent five hours reading about the incarnation of Christ from the viewpoints of Karl Barth and Thomas Aquinas. I reckon I grasped about 10 per cent of it. I learnt some new words, though. 'Ontological' was one.

I met Lee's new son Zach Joseph for the first time. We'd always fantasized about taking our boys on all sorts of adventures. Now it could happen. Anna's nesting has reached epic proportions. There's nothing left for her to clean or tidy away. Except me.

Monday 8 November

The orthodontist says it will cost thousands to get my teeth straightened. I can't justify it. Not with Mum paying. I'm also not sure how I feel about cosmetic surgery. Joel Wood listened to my concerns. He sent me this scripture from Isaiah 53.2: 'He hath no form or comeliness: and when we see him, there is no beauty that we should desire him.' That's it then. I can live with crooked teeth. Mum was so relieved! Probing a bit deeper, it turns out that she only wanted to do it in the first place because of some of her parental insecurities. She wept as I reassured her that she always did her best. 'You don't need to get my teeth straightened to prove how much you've loved me, Mum,' I said. The consultation she paid for has already led me to finally stop sucking my thumb. Result.

Thursday 11 November

I'm inspired afresh to live fuller and deeper after reading this cracking extract from Shakespeare's *Julius Caesar*:

Cowards die many times before their deaths;
The valiant never taste of death but once.
Of all the wonders that I have yet heard,
It seems to me most strange that men should fear;
Seeing that death, a necessary end,
Will come when it will come.

The promise of eternity with Christ should inform every part of my life now. So why am I so full of restlessness, fear and insecurity?

Friday 12 November

Anna and I have just watched *The Social Network*. Like good citizens of Yorkshire, we sneaked our own popcorn in because of the crazy cinema prices. The auditorium was deserted so I made Anna laugh by running to the front to dance. The film gave a fascinating insight into human relationships. For all his success, drive and creativity, all Mark Zuckerberg really seemed to crave was love and acceptance. How ironic that Facebook connected people in more ways than ever before and yet destroyed the friendship of the two young lads who created it. It's a parable.

I'm doing an essay on the origins and liturgy of the Anglican ordination service. It's driving home the enormity of what I'm about to do with my life. The 1552 version has the bishop say: 'Take heed that the persons, whom ye present unto us, be apt and meet, for their learning and godly conversation, to exercise their ministry, duly, to the honour of God, and the edifying of his church.' I don't feel ready or worthy yet to be that person.

Saturday 13 November

Amazing session with Sister Cecilia this morning at the Bede Centre. She's so affirming. I'm so relieved that she's agreed to be my spiritual director up to ordination and beyond. Doing life and faith without my beloved nun would leave me bereft.

I tried out another one of her St Ignatius-inspired spiritual exercises today. She gently invited me to close my eyes, quieten my mind and imagine being physically present with God. 'Where are you, Matt?' she asked after a while. A clear picture gradually emerged of Jesus and I walking and talking along a dusty road. We were just like two close friends, easy in each other's company, jawing about nothing in particular. 'What picture best describes who you are right now, Matt?' Cecilia probed. Immediately the image of a firework came to mind. Some exploded into the night sky, bringing whoops of joy from a gathered crowd. Other rockets sputtered out before catching light. 'Where are you and Jesus now, Matt?' We were sitting on soft hay in the back of a rickety, slow moving cart. Boxes of fireworks were stacked all around us. It was so peaceful. The air was warm, the sun beginning to go down. Jesus was smiling at me. We talked quietly. The cart gently rocked us. I was struck by the powerful sense that there was nothing urgent we had to do. There was no particular place we had to get to, or fireworks we had to light. It was just me and Jesus relaxed and happy together in the back of that slow-moving cart. I didn't want to be parted from him. I was safe. At peace. Content.

Eventually, Sister Cecilia gently brought me back to reality. An hour had passed in what felt like a minute. She didn't try to analyse or dissect my picture. She simply said it was my gift to draw from. 'Keep going back to it, Matt. Just you and Jesus in the back of that cart.' Nuns are the best.

In the most extreme gear change to any day I can remember recently, hours after leaving the convent I was sat round a table playing poker with Dan 'the tan' Adams and the boys. And yet, between hands, in the midst of the banter, beer and industrial language, the conversation was all about God. They all had a view.

Nick is fascinated by faith but doesn't believe because of the suffering in the world. Dom is dragged along to his partner's church some Sundays but doesn't really get it yet. Charlie loves the Christian values and is determined to bring his daughter up to adhere to them. But he struggles with faith. He doubts the miracles and supernatural accounts of Christ's life. Eric admitted that he'd seen inmates at the prison where he works be transformed by God. Dan was cagey and evasive. I sat enthralled by their honesty and openness. Six boozy lads talking about faith and God round a poker table for two hours. From the convent to the poker table, God is working everywhere. And he lets me join in.

Wednesday 17 November

I knelt at the tomb of St Cuthbert in Durham Cathedral with Mum and Grandma to pray for Aunty Lynne. It was a holy moment. We each lit a candle for her. Later on Mum bought me a cheap shirt from Oxfam Boutique and the new Take That CD for herself. 'I want to support them,' she said. 'Support them? Mum, they're millionaire pop stars!' I said. 'But they're such nice lads, Matt.' Nutter.

Friday 19 November

Sleep is so fleeting. I keep imagining Anna screaming out that her waters have broken. It could happen tonight.

Monday 22 November

I was horrible to Anna this morning. I was horrible to Paul Bromley this afternoon. Peace is now restored with both of them but I still feel wretched. Anna was snoring too loudly next to me in bed as I tried to write a letter. I barked at her to be quiet and attempted to roll her into a less cacophonous position. It didn't go down well. She stormed downstairs. I eventually got her back into bed after a grovelling apology.

I'm learning that there's just some people you should never try to stop snoring. Your heavily pregnant wife is definitely one of them. I got back to Durham in a foul, uncooperative mood. Paul was caught in the crossfire. I snapped that it was always me helping him with essays and feeding him the right books. 'It's all one way traffic, Paul!' I growled. He just rolled his eyes and left me to it. I'm such a toad.

Our systematics lecturer flapped like a seal in a swimming pool during a discussion about who God is. It's a common problem here. Our theological teachers and guides will not – or perhaps cannot – ever give a definitive answer about anything. It seems we are called as priests to believe and minister in a state of perpetual mystery when it comes to the nature of God. I texted my old boss Reverend John during the lecture: 'Who is God?' He replied, simply: '?' I texted back: 'Exactly'. Pre-Cranmer it all used to be so straightforward.

At her scan today, the doctors told Anna that both of the twins weighed 5lb 7oz. The induction date is 6 December.

Wednesday 24 November

I led our discipleship group session this morning. Using *Amazing Grace* as inspiration, I got them to reflect on 'the hour they first believed'. One of the challenges of college life, I said, is that we can easily lose our child-like faith in Jesus because of all the essays, debate and questions. There's a danger we become cynical, and view faith as an academic exercise rather than a supernatural relationship with the Living God. I encouraged the group to cling onto the truth of that hour of first belief. Everything else flows out of it.

I met Harry for another placement session. Surely it's not supposed to be this much fun? We're thrilled that my press release about the work of Sally and her estate team appeared in the *Northern Echo*. I hope it does some good.

Thursday 25 November

As I write this, Aunty Lynne is not expected to survive the night. She collapsed in Tesco and has internal bleeding. Jo doesn't land from Doha until 10 a.m. tomorrow. We're all praying she makes it in time to say goodbye to her mum. What a flight that must be. Cancer is the cruellest disease.

I've spent a lot of time thinking about Aunty Lynne tonight. She has been a towering figure in my life. Amy and I spent half our childhood eating her casseroles to escape Dad's oppressive moods. I hope she's aware of the depth of our love and gratitude. I may not get the chance to tell her again. Amy phoned me in tears. She's spoken to Becky and Lorrie. Apparently Aunty Lynne keeps telling them to 'Look after Ally' over and over again.

The pain of death. The beauty of new life. We're seeing it all as a family. In the time two lives have grown within Anna's womb, Aunty Lynne's body has degenerated to such a degree that she's now on the brink of death. Anna could give birth in one ward at York Hospital while Aunty Lynne is dying in another one. She may already have slipped away as I write this. I can't get my head round it all. Lord, have mercy. We prayed for her during Night Prayer tonight. Paul tried to lift my spirits. We watched a dodgy action film in his room. He brought me Monster Munch and a Curly Wurly. What a beautiful man.

Friday 26 November

Aunty Lynne has survived another day. What a relief that Jo made it back to be with her. Uncle Ally has taken the decision to bring her home. She's now on a drip in her beloved front room. Ally and the girls are keeping vigil beside the sofa.

It's wonderful to be back in Anna's arms. We're struggling to get excited about the babies when the family we love are in so much pain.

Saturday 27 November

Aunty Lynne can't face any visitors except Ally and the girls so a few of us gathered at Mum's. We shared our feelings over copious amounts of tea and Rocky bars. It's frustrating not being able to do anything to help. Grandma went round to see Aunty Lynne briefly. She described her as frail and thin but alert. 'Lynne wanted me to stay and have a sandwich like I always do,' she said.

Anna and I gathered in the nursery in the early hours. We couldn't sleep. We watched the snow come down in clumps and settle on the garden. The moment was bittersweet. Bitter as we thought about Aunty Lynne lying on that sofa; sweet as we imagined the babies asleep in this room. We'll miss our home when we move to Hull. It's safe and warm and familiar. It's part of us. It was always Anna's dream to live here.

Sunday 28 November

It's one drama after another right now. Dad called from Berlin. He's been helping my godfather Chris research his new book. I could instantly tell something was up. Apparently he found Chris dead in his hotel bed. He'd suffered a heart attack. Chris was one of my journalistic heroes growing up. He'd always bring me back awesome souvenirs from his travels covering sport around the world for the *Daily Express*. He once sent me Ayrton Senna's autograph. Chris had become an authority on East Germany and the collapse of the Berlin wall. Dad had a haunted sound in his voice. He's making the arrangements to bring his body back.

I spoke to Aunty Lynne on the phone this morning. I was busy talking to people at church when Mum suddenly thrust me the phone. Aunty Lynne was shouting 'hello' in that funny voice she does. She then said: 'I'm still here, Matt! I'm not dead yet!' Talk about lifting the tension. I said how much I loved her. What a gift to get that opportunity. Jo later told me a wonderful story about a colleague from her school in Doha. This lady paid out of her own pocket to fly back to the UK so Jo wasn't on her own on that horrible flight. She then got a plane straight back to Doha. What Christlikeness. Sometimes human beings just make your heart sing.

Wednesday 1 December

Our neighbour Frank has taught me a valuable lesson about what it means to serve others. Gazing out of my office window yesterday, I noticed that Frank's next-door neighbour Dave had cleared his own drive of snow but no one else's. I remember thinking that it was a bit selfish he didn't clear Frank's too. Today I watched Frank as he got up and not only cleared his own drive but Dave's as well. He then crossed the street and cleared our drive. That's servanthood.

I expressed to Anna and her mum how much this gesture had really touched me. They both pointed out that I had sat happy and warm watching from the window as Frank cleared all that snow on his own. Surely the right thing to do was to go out and help him? Fair point.

Thursday 2 December

I cleared some drives of snow today.

Saturday 4 December

Aunty Lynne continues to fight on. I met up with Uncle Mike at Mum's house. We compiled our top five Bob Dylan songs. 'Girl from the North Country', 'Sad-Eyed Lady of the Lowlands' and 'Don't Think Twice, It's All Right' all made the cut. Dad has agreed to take me to Auschwitz at the end of March. I want to try to get my head round what happened there before I get ordained.

Monday 6 December

Ecclesiastes 3.1–2 articulates this day better than I could. It's midnight. We've been in a room at York Hospital all day waiting for the babies to be born. Anna is in agony, moving back and forth on top of a giant birth ball. It actually looks quite comical but I daren't tell her that.

Aunty Lynne has finally succumbed to her cancer. She died at 4.30 a.m.: 'There is a time for everything … A time to be born, and a time to die.' Mum broke the news to me at 7 a.m. I briefly spoke to Jo on the phone. She's relieved but profoundly sad. Uncle Ally and the girls were beside her in the front room for eleven days. Jo said it was Aunty Lynne's wish that I take the funeral. Jo will give a eulogy. What a privilege.

I visited them in Beech Grove before taking Anna to the hospital to start the inducing. Arriving at the door, I was suddenly conscious of the familiarity of this home. How it makes me feel so safe. The love I always found inside. Uncle Ally greeted me in the porch. His eyes were puffy and red. It's the first time I've seen him look small, and helpless. Grief does that, I suppose. We embraced. I reassured him that I'd take care of the funeral service. He just kept repeating that it was our time now.

We got to the hospital and settled in a comfortable room. Anna was uptight. Nothing really happened for the first few hours. She was hooked up to a machine that monitored the babies' heartbeats. Whatever a cervix is or does, gel kept being smothered into it. I'm guessing it's the babies' route out of Anna and into the world. We were eventually allowed out to go for a coffee in the hospital café. Jonny and Anne were in there. Anne's dad Alf had a serious stroke this morning. Jonny was bitten by a dog yesterday and needed a tetanus jab.

I later spent an hour in the chapel asking God to help me make sense of it all. I wrote some memories and thoughts down about Aunty Lynne. Anna had more gel inserted into her. The pain is excruciating, apparently. Watching was painful enough. 'I've got hold of your cervix, Anna', our midwife Pam said, as calmly as if she'd just passed her a custard cream. It reassures me that they do this stuff dozens of times a day. At one point, Pam called on me to help get the next dose of gel out because one of her hands was literally inside Anna. I clumsily pressed too hard on the sachet and it squirted everywhere. Anna laughed. Pam didn't.

So here we are. A time to be born. A time to die. What a crazy, sad, happy, weird day. Thank you, God, for Aunty Lynne. For her love and generosity. For her lust for life and family and sunny holidays. Please bless us with two healthy babies. Amen.

It's 12.30 p.m. now. Anna has vacated the birth ball and is now on all fours, sucking in air like it's her last breath. I should really stop writing this and rub her back or something.

Tuesday 7 December

Esther Rose and Heidi Mae finally came into the world at 3.20 p.m. and 3.41 p.m. Esther weighed 5lb 7oz, Heidi 5lb 10oz. Our midwife Emily was a constant reassuring and helpful presence. No verse of profound poetry could properly express how it felt to finally hold them. All that waiting. All that longing. All that being told it could never happen. Gone. I'll hold Esther and Heidi countless times in their lives – whether they like it or not. But nothing will ever match this first time. It was like holding hope.

The day had started badly. From the early hours onwards, Anna's pain intensified. Her screaming reached hideous levels. I felt so helpless and afraid. Inevitably I kept saying the wrong thing. 'How do you feel?' I asked feebly at one point. *'How do you think I feel?!!'* Anna shouted back, only with more f-words. We tried everything to ease the pain: hot baths, rolling on a birth ball, crouching, pacing, lying down, standing up. Nothing worked. I was on the verge of delirium by the end. Anna was in bad shape too.

In the midst of all this, I got a text from Uncle Mike to say Debbie's dad Eric had died. He was a lovely man. They all called him 'The Maestro'. The human drama wheel keeps turning.

So this is how it finally happened. We were ushered into the labour ward at about 10.30 a.m. Anna was injected with an epidural, put in the labour position, and told to push. After an hour of this no heads had emerged. Anna was taken into theatre, and they brought in the big guns. Serious-looking medical instruments were put into the hands of what seemed like about 15 unsmiling medics. Just get them out alive, I thought. Just get them out alive. I made the decision to stay head-end throughout. The risks to our future love-making were too great. I don't remember much about the doctor who pulled Esther out with forceps, except that she had hair like Seve Ballesteros.

It's funny what comes to mind in moments of high stress and emotion. My daughter was suddenly just there. Alive and purple. A human life that we'd made had come out of my wife! And just like that I was a dad. A father. Papa. An indescribable love coursed through me as I looked down on her face. But there was more to come. One more. Esther and I sat ringside as they struggled to get her sister out. The situation got serious very quickly. Heidi's arm was tucked behind her head making the exit out of Anna's innards tricky. Her heart rate was dropping. The scalpels were poised for a Caesarean. They focused Anna for one last effort. She pushed and heaved with a new urgency. Dr Seve wrenched and pulled with the forceps. She did it. Heidi came out. She took her first breath of the world's air before being whisked away for tests. Such relief! Anna cried out: 'I didn't give you a boy!' It hadn't even registered. I'm all about the girls now.

The rest of the night is a blur. We were left alone in the recovery room for a precious hour before the hordes arrived. I looked deep into Anna's tired, happy eyes and expressed my love and gratitude.

I couldn't stop thinking about the GP who told me that we'd be forever childless. It's worth recording again what he actually said: 'If I was a betting man, Mr Woodcock, I'd never put money on you being a father.' But anything is possible with God. Anything. We held hands as I thanked him in prayer for our sleeping daughters. We are parents! I left my girls to sleep.

There was one job left to do: wetting the girls' heads with my mates in the Fox. At last I could join in with their stories about the trials of being a dad. I got home and wrote a letter to the Cranmer community, thanking them for their love and prayers. It's also Mum's birthday today. How lovely. Anna still remembered to get her a card from us. Two grandchildren wasn't a bad present either. I'm in bed writing this as a father of two girls. Oh crap! Thank you, God.

Wednesday 8 December

My first full day as a dad. Anna was in bits when I arrived at the hospital. She'd only managed two hours' sleep. Esther keeps barfing up womb mucus. She retches and gags and looks like she's choking to death. I couldn't watch. I'm responsible for this little thing now but I don't have a clue what to do. My stress caused Anna stress. We are floundering. Who teaches you to do this stuff? I need someone on permanent standby to reassure us.

Debbie has asked me to take her dad's funeral. It's a strange time of light and shade for our family. We are mourning the loss of two precious lives and celebrating the birth of two new ones. And I am front and centre of both. Talk about a life of extremes. I fled Esther's barfs to sort out Aunty Lynne's funeral service with Jo, Lorrie and Uncle Ally. It was important to her that I took it. When Jo said it might be too much for me, Aunty Lynne replied: 'Well, ask him to try.' I can hear her saying it. Jo has written a beautiful eulogy. It says:

I asked Mum if there was anything that she wanted me to particularly say, or any message that she would like to give. She said this: 'Just tell everyone, "Thank you for their love and support over the years and tell them there is not one day of my life that I regret or that I would change. I've had the best life ever and loved every minute."' Things that remind me of Mum: holidays; wonderful cooking; cricket teas; her bike; Marks & Spencer; Cava; Scrabble.

The funeral director presumed I was an old hand at funerals. He asked me: 'Where do you want the commendation in the order of service, Matt?' I'm thinking, 'What's a commendation?' I think I convinced them that I sort of know what I'm doing.

We were inundated with visitors at the hospital this afternoon. Mike, Rose, Hannah, Sarah, Rob, Elsie, Thomas, Amy, Phoebe, Honor, Mum, Grandma – it was brilliant chaos! I met Dad later in the Hole in the Wall. The babies' heads needed more wetting. Topics for discussion included our Auschwitz trip, Franz Klammer's famous final run in the Olympic downhill skiing and the war photographs of Dad's friend, Tom Stoddart. Tears leaked out when I got home. Sitting in the front room, all I could think about was how helpless I felt when Esther cried and retched. I am so responsible. I suspect I was unconsciously crying away my old life. It will never be the same again.

Thursday 9 December

I keep catching myself with a stupid smile on my face. I changed Heidi's nappy for the first time this morning. Her poo was black.

Friday 10 December

Esther's screams go right through me. They're unbearable. I'm a nervous wreck. At the slightest murmur from the Moses basket,

I run in to roll a glass against their bare legs to check for meningitis. I panic when they move too much. I panic when they're too still. I stupidly even asked the midwife if she thought Esther had Down's Syndrome. 'Of course not!' the midwife replied. 'Why would you ask that?' 'Because I'm terrified, that's why!' I wanted to shout back. 'Just tell me they're going to be healthy and happy for the rest of their lives!' Out of the two of them, Heidi is far easier. She lies there still and serene.

Anna's post-pregnancy hormone frenzy has kicked in. We were told to expect it after about three days. She can't stop crying. She thinks she's a rubbish mum. It got so bad last night that she fantasized about being childless again. The feeling quickly passed but she cried all night because of the guilt of even thinking it. Amy and Mum were our salvation tonight. They came to the ward room with encouragement and reassurance. And wine. Lots and lots of wine. Anna unloaded all her fears and frustrations. We listened, between sips. Lots and lots of sips.

Saturday 11 December

We've brought the babies home. I keep praying for God's peace. Surely there comes a time when you become immune to your own children's cries and even begin to find them endearing? Any time soon would be good. We took Esther and Heidi to see Uncle Ally. We hoped it would give him a lift. He cradled them in his big bricklayer arms.

I sorted out Eric's funeral with his family this afternoon. They sat in his front room and shared their favourite memories. Eric's three daughters will all pay tribute. I'm not sure if he believed in God. Debbie said he went to church with them sometimes. The tea and biscuits at the end were his favourite bit. Maybe there was more going on that kept drawing him back? Esther has just started crying again. It's going to be a long night.

Sunday 12 December

We've just endured one of the hardest nights of our marriage. The babies refused to settle. Every time we put them into their basket they screamed. Every time we picked them back up they stopped. At about 4 a.m. I had hold of Esther and Anna had hold of Heidi. We caught each other's weary gaze. A moment of clarity passed between us that went beyond words. This is what we had longed and prayed for. We can do this. Sue came to our rescue at 8 a.m. Anna crumpled emotionally when she walked in. They had a mother and daughter moment. Anne Wooldridge came round and Anna cried in her arms. Anne then wept when we asked her to be Heidi's godmother. It's one big sob-fest after another.

The real saviour of the day was Debbie's niece Emma. If we never see her again she'll always occupy a special place in our hearts. Her presence felt like a gift from God. She came round after hearing about Anna's struggles to get Esther to breastfeed. Emma is a trained midwife who exudes authority and strength. Her first words to Anna were: 'I'm not leaving this house until you can do it!' She kept her word. It took hours. But Emma would not give up until Esther was suckling properly. She used an array of techniques but the one that really worked was to literally push Esther's face right into the breast. What joy to see her finally hoovering up big milky gulps.

Anna can feed both girls at once using a special shelf-like contraption. The house now resembles a dairy farm. I've decided that this day will be forever dedicated to Saint Emma – patron saint of breastfeeding. She's made my wife extremely happy. Hormonal with scabby red nipples, but very, very happy.

Monday 13 December

I commended Aunty Lynne to God at York Crematorium today. A wonderful serenity possessed me as I looked out on all the grieving people. This is my calling. My privilege. 'God was with her in life, and he's still with her now,' I said. I was encouraged throughout by a beautiful framed photograph of Aunty Lynne placed on top of her coffin. I glanced at it for inspiration. It's a picture of vitality and flourishing. That was Aunty Lynne. I couldn't look at Uncle Ally. At the end of the service, I laid my hands on the coffin to say the words of commendation: 'We entrust Aunty Lynne to your mercy in the name of Jesus our Lord'. Harry Nilsson sang us out. It finished everyone off. Is there a more distressing lyric in pop than, 'I can't live, if living is without you'?

We packed out the Marcia for the wake. It buzzed with laughter, reminiscences and glasses of Cava being filled to the brim. The fragrance of Aunty Lynne was everywhere. Jo, Becky and Lorrie had drenched themselves in her favourite perfume. It was after midnight by the time Jo and I walked Uncle Ally home through the ice and snow. We linked arms and staggered and slid down Beech Grove, laughing and crying and remembering.

Wednesday 15 December

Anna is a feeding machine. Esther and Heidi can't get enough of her breast-fresh milk. A wave of jealousy swept over me as I watched them greedily guzzle on her bosoms. The bosoms that were once mine alone to enjoy. I resisted the urge to shout: 'My turn!' I'm trying to stay focused on keeping Anna operational with cups of tea, words of encouragement and plumped-up cushions. Previously, I'd never plumped up a cushion in my life. I wonder when we can start making love again? Is it too soon to mention it? What's a reasonable timescale?

Thursday 16 December

I had the pleasure of taking Eric 'The Maestro' Hinchcliffe's funeral today. It didn't all run smoothly. Minutes before his coffin arrived, I made the mistake of taking my script into the toilet. I splashed water all over it while washing my hands. It smudged the words and I was forced to do a frantic rewrite from memory. It wasn't the greatest preparation. The chapel was packed as I led the coffin in to 'My Way'. Eric was a huge Sinatra fan. Then the first hymn happened. I announced that we'd stand to sing 'The Lord's My Shepherd'. Glancing over to the organ, my insides liquefied. The seat was empty. No organist. He hadn't turned up.

The crematorium warden made the 'cut it' sign across his neck as he nervously paced at the back. Taking a deep breath, I said: 'I'm really sorry, ladies and gentlemen, but it appears that the organist hasn't turned up. I've forgotten the tune to this hymn – does anyone know it?' Complete silence. After what felt like days, Debbie suddenly began to sing. A few others joined in. Then some more. Before long the whole place was going for it. What a moment! 'You can always rely on Debbie,' I said after it had finished. 'Your dad would have been proud.'

Friday 17 December

Ian has just texted to tell me his mum has died. Phyllis was a formidable woman. What I call a 'proper' Christian. She was relentless in trying to do good. It's nice to see Ian's biting humour is still intact. He texted: 'You'll be pleased to know that my mam's dying wish was that under no circumstances should you lead the funeral.'

Mike Laycock came to interview us about Esther and Heidi for the *Press*. It was weird to be on the other side of the notebook. It gave us an opportunity to speak out over the IVF postcode lottery. If you live in York, it costs thousands of pounds to get the treatment. If you live in Hull or Leeds you can get IVF free on the NHS. That can't be fair. So many poor couples are being deprived the chance of having kids just because they live in the 'wrong' city.

It was nine months ago that the Cranmer community prayed in the chapel for a miracle. Now we have two of them upstairs. And they are screaming. Loudly.

Saturday 18 December

Endured another worry-filled sleepless night. This time I'd convinced myself that Esther's heavy breathing was severe asthma or cystic fibrosis. I've got to relax.

Monday 20 December

I've stumbled upon a wonderful John Betjeman poem called 'The Conversion of St Paul'. He talks about stumbling on and blindly groping, but being 'upheld by intermittent hope'. I know exactly what he means. That's my truth.

I sat with Ian tonight so he could offload about losing his mum. He shared what she meant to him, and some regrets he still had. He was refreshingly candid for once. I reassured him that his mum died knowing with absolute certainty that he loved her. And he lives on knowing that she loved him. Sometimes that's all we can ask for.

We ended up watching *Ghostbusters* with a Chinese. It annoyed me that Ian's chicken in black bean sauce was far superior to my special fried rice. First world problems.

Tuesday 21 December

I heard a hilarious story about Pastor Bob today. He was thanking God for us during the Galtres Church carol concert. At one point he said: 'Thank you, Lord, that you healed Woody of his impotence and blessed them with Esther and Heidi.' Apparently the whole church descended into fits of laughter. I've texted this to Bob to put him straight: 'Stop telling people I'm impotent! I'm infertile – it's a very big difference!'

Friday 24 December

We were front-page news today. The *Press* splashed with our 'Christmas miracles' story. It felt so strange after years trying to get on the front with a story I'd written. Now I was being written about. They used a cute picture of Esther and Heidi inside two Christmas stockings. The headline said: '"The best presents we could wish for": IVF couple beat all the odds to welcome their Christmas miracles.' I'm now unofficially the *Press* spokesman for men with low sperm counts.

Inside it read: 'New dad Matt said he wanted to help break the taboo surrounding male infertility. He said some men had a hang-up about having a low sperm count, but it was a growing problem and nothing to be embarrassed or ashamed about.' I received some lovely messages about the story. Old friends and colleagues came out of the woodwork to get in touch. An old *Press* colleague quipped: 'That's the best story with your name on I've ever seen on page one of the *Press*! Better than "Acomb woman's wheelie bin fury" or whatever guff you used to churn out.' Fair comment.

Saturday 25 December

Our first Christmas Day as a family of four. Anna's face was beautiful when she opened her new mini-laptop. I was delighted with my big bag of Refresher sweets, *Desire* by Bob Dylan and *Mad Men* Season 3. The St Paul's service was packed.

I met the gang as usual in the Fox. Lee and I exchanged gifts. Paul and Sue bought me a tyre pump. We played Wii Sports all night in their front room. The red wine didn't help my coordination. Great day.

Sunday 26 December

Aunty Lynne was never far from our thoughts today. It was sad and weird not being at their Boxing Day party. To not walk into that warm, familiar home to be greeted by piles of wonderful food, a big cheer and Uncle Ally telling me to help myself to the beer-can mountain.

Amy hosted her first family party this afternoon. Keith did a quiz. We all struggled to spell 'Rhododendron'. I got home and spent a long time just looking at Esther and Heidi. Then they started crying.

Monday 27 December

Dad has bought me *Schindler's Ark* to read and Górecki's Third Symphony to listen to in preparation for our trip to Auschwitz. It's a beautiful, haunting piece of music. Rachmaninov's Piano Concerto No. 2, Nick Drake's *Five Leaves Left* and early Bob Dylan are my usual soundtrack to the dark times. Now I can add Górecki. The second movement is inspired by a lady's short prayer found on the wall of Cell No. 3 in the Gestapo headquarters in Zakopane. The writer begs the Virgin Mary not to desert her in her hour of need. Dad accompanied the gifts with a note. It said: 'If you're in the right mood and receptive, the work [Górecki] will break your heart. With the book, too, I think you'll be ready emotionally for Auschwitz.' I'm actually quite apprehensive about the trip. It's often cited as proof against the existence of God. A place where the birds don't sing. My faith is rooted in hope. What if I don't find any in Auschwitz?

Tuesday 28 December

I'm reading a fascinating book by Andrew Roberts, *Hitler and Churchill: Secrets of Leadership*. It's packed full of wisdom and great quotes. I love this extract from a Churchill radio broadcast at the height of the Second World War:

It is a message of good cheer to our fighting forces … They know that they have behind them a people who will not flinch or

weary of the struggle – hard and protracted though it will be;
but that we shall rather draw from the heart of suffering itself
the means of inspiration and survival, and of victory won not
for ourselves but for all – a victory not only for our own time,
but for the long and better days that are to come.

I can only imagine how stirring that was to hear live on the radio as an ordinary family.

Roberts articulates wonderfully the key difference between how Churchill and Hitler impacted and inspired those around them. It's an important lesson for every church leader to learn. He writes: 'After meeting Hitler people felt that he, the Führer, could achieve anything. But when people met Churchill they felt that they themselves could achieve anything.' I could do with some of that gift in a church context. Those flowers won't arrange themselves.

Wednesday 29 December

I watched the darts tonight at Keith and Amy's. It's such an exciting sport. Sid Waddell is one of our country's great orators. His best line tonight was: 'He's only had a shandy but he could go home legless.' Magic darts.

Friday 31 December

This has probably been my most significant year to date. I read back and reflected on some of its key days. Days of darkness and doubt. Days of promise and joy. Days of life and death. My love for Anna has grown deeper. We shouldn't work, really. We're so different. She has carried so much emotionally and physically. I'll always remember this year for the faith of those around me. When mine faltered, when God seemed distant and cold, they strengthened me. People with big faith pray big prayers. They pray for miracles – and believe they're possible.

My last hours of the year were spent trying to cope with Esther's nerve-shredding cries. How appropriate. We saw in the New Year at Mum's. She'd received a lovely letter from Ronnie, expressing his joy at the jumper she sent and the photos of Esther and Heidi. He has such literary flair. 'I celebrate with you all, new small souls into your family, twins with beautiful features and names.' We watched *The Karate Kid* and toasted the memory of Aunty Lynne. I'm full of hope for the New Year. Always hope.

Year Three

Sunday 2 January

I attended the 8.45 a.m. service at St Paul's. Tom Charles preached on the Epiphany. He loves to wrestle with and question the eternal truths of God. He tried to unpack the complexity and mystery of the incarnation and the difficulties in answering the question, who is Jesus? Tom got quite defensive when I chatted to him afterwards. 'Well, I'm not evangelical, I'm a liberal,' he said. 'My daughter-in-law is a Muslim.' I wanted to snap back: 'Well, I'm a Christian and my best mate's a butcher. So what?' Labels annoy me.

I've written a letter to Jo's colleague in Doha. She was the one who accompanied her on the flight back to the UK when Aunty Lynne collapsed. I thanked her on behalf of the family. It was an act of kindness that has inspired us all. She's called Teresa Woulfe. It's a name to remember. I feel sure she'll crop up in a sermon one day.

Tuesday 4 January

I was inspired tonight by Sister Mary Nirmala. She was the woman who took on the almost impossible task of following in the footsteps of Mother Teresa as head of the Missionaries of Charity. Asked by a journalist how she coped with that burden, she replied: 'If I think of myself I am frightened, but if I look at God, at his love and entrust myself to his prayer, I think I will manage.'

Friday 7 January

Esther's weight has rocketed to nearly 8lb. The health visitor said Anna's breast milk was like gold top.

I love the encounter between Oskar Schindler and Itzhak Stern in *Schindler's Ark* where they discuss the possibility of a loving, caring God in light of the Nazi horrors. Schindler sympathizes with the priests who had to keep telling people that if he cared about the death of a single sparrow how much more would he care about them. 'Stern agreed but suggested, in the spirit of the discussion, that the

Bible reference Herr Schindler had made could be summed up by a Talmudic verse which said that he who saves the life of one man, saves the entire world.' I'll be using that in a sermon.

My future boss, Neal, has been in the *Hull Daily Mail* twice recently. The first story was about them giving people the 'wow' factor when they walk into Holy Trinity. Today's story is about them losing £1,000 a week. What worries me is that both stories are about the building. What about the people? I said I wanted a challenge.

Tuesday 11 January

Proverbs 23.31–33, says:

> *Do not gaze at wine when it's red*
> *when it sparkles in the cup,*
> *when it goes down smoothly!*
> *In the end it bites like a snake*
> *and poisons like a viper.*
> *Your eyes will see strange sights,*
> *and your mind will imagine confusing things.*

Reading it in a modern context, it could also have added: 'And you will send ridiculous, judgemental text messages to your closest friends and make a complete fool of yourself.'

Yes, I had a drink last night for the first time in ages. In the haze of red wine enlightenment, I decided to put a few of the lads right about some things. I told Lee that it was time to stop messing God around and take him seriously. I implored Ian to get back involved in a church. I remonstrated with Aidan about something (it turns out) he didn't actually do. I also texted Pete that I loved him like a brother. No wonder Lee calls me 'The Cringe'. I really am. I'm done with the red wine viper.

I'm obsessed with *Mad Men*. Like all great anti-heroes, Don Draper is maddeningly complex. He has the American Dream in the palm of his hand but he can't cope with it. He's too hard-wired to self-destruction. No matter how much business success he has, women he sleeps with or whisky he drinks, Don can't find peace. He's a walking parable.

I emailed my tutor Stuart to tell him about Holy Trinity's financial troubles. I wanted to encourage him that his seminars were brilliant preparation for me. Teaching us lot can be a deadening experience at times I guess. It's nice for them to know that some of it might actually be relevant. Stuart replied in typically spiritual fashion:

> *Big hill to climb but nothing's impossible for God … If you and your boss focus on building the Kingdom the money will follow. My lectures won't prepare you (maybe a little bit). Prayer and prayer and more prayer will prepare you.*

I took the babies for a walk into Acomb this afternoon. A host of familiar faces honked and waved. Local property tycoon Ian Thornley was one. He shouted over: 'Good job they aren't boys, Woody – we don't need two more like you!' Thanks, Ian.

Wednesday 12 January

I'm fascinated to know how Esther and Heidi's personalities will develop. What will they sound like? What will interest them? What will their favourite food be? I'm already worried about them meeting boys. If I'm dead, girls, and you're reading this, convent life is not as bad as it sounds. Boys are the enemy. Don't believe anything they say. Don't give them anything they want. Ever.

Sunday 16 January

It was the worst goodbye ever tonight. Leaving my girls to drive back to Durham was horrendous. I held Esther and Heidi in turn, praying for God's protection over them. Smothering their faces with kisses, I told them to look after Mummy. Then I cried with Anna on the doorstep. I feel so guilty knowing that she'll be feeding the girls through the night. The last time I slept in my college bed, Aunty Lynne was alive and we were childless. How quickly the seasons of life change.

Thursday 20 January

Poor Paul Bromley. Being nearest to me in college, he yet again felt the full force of my morning moodiness. I was so unnecessarily critical of his reading of the lesson at Morning Prayer. He looked crestfallen. It got worse. Grumping my way into the common room to make a brew, lovely Liam came bounding up to me like a panting Labrador. He wanted a quiet word. 'I'm in a bad mood,' I barked, 'I need a cup of tea. Talk to me later.' It was beyond rude even for me. I eventually found Liam to apologize and see what he wanted. He said: 'All I wanted to let you know, Matt, is that I've been praying for you and your future ministry at Holy Trinity every day on my way to college. It's on my heart to commit to keep doing it until you leave. I just wanted to let you know.' I don't possess the words to describe how bad and convicted I felt in that moment. The people here are too nice for me. I don't deserve them.

Our New Testament lecturer was on fire today. It was our first session on the Gospel of John. He is a gifted, wise, irascible, opinionated teacher who I've grown to grudgingly admire. He talked about John's Gospel being shallow enough for a baby to paddle in but deep enough to drown an elephant. If you think you've grasped the book, we were warned, you haven't. You never will. I'm daunted but excited at the prospect of plunging John's depths.

Friday 21 January

My girls have grown and developed in the space of a week. Anna has relented and let Heidi suck a dummy, such is her agitation and restlessness at night.

Our pioneer ministry seminar was tense and difficult. There was a lot of passionate disagreement. Aidan lost it with me because he didn't feel I was letting him get his point across. That's not easy to do with Aidan. He shouted: *'No, Matt Woodcock!'* at the top of his voice. There was something of a Mexican standoff between us. Aidan later texted to say he loved me with an 'unquenchable passion' and asked for forgiveness. I texted back to say I granted him my absolution.

Monday 24 January

Ecclesiastes is dominating my life at the moment as I try to finish my 4,000-word Old Testament essay. It's a fascinating, perplexing book that speaks profoundly into the reality of today's world. The author seems to be having some sort of nervous breakdown. He's rich and successful but unfulfilled. He's a mass of contradictions. The pursuit of wealth and carnal pleasure doesn't fulfil him, but then he writes: 'Feasts are made for laughter; wine gladdens life, and money meets every need.' I was drawn to this observation he makes about the dead: '… never again will they have any share in all that happens under the sun'. I have the hope of heaven, but until I get there, I want to fully share in and contribute to what happens under the sun. Starting tomorrow.

Wednesday 26 January

I'm a deeply unpleasant, insecure man at times. Too often lately I've indulged my hungry ego with titbits. Today I found myself engineering conversations so I could let people know that I got 87 per cent in my preaching assessment. I was desperate for them to know. This is not priestly behaviour.

If Paul Bromley and I are the future of the Church of England then it's really in trouble. I joined him in his room at midnight after an intense night of study. We drank port and listened to Iron Maiden. How and why I don't know, but before long we'd typed 'Farting newsreaders' into YouTube. Tears rolled down our cheeks as we watched a Scandinavian news anchor trump while reading the bulletin. She tried to blame her chair before collapsing into hysterics. I can still hear Paul belly laughing himself to sleep next door.

Thursday 27 January

To mark Holocaust Memorial Day, Joel and I gathered in the chapel to pray and reflect. We read extracts from *Schindler's Ark*.

Laurie asked a few of us to pray for him tonight about his inability to resist sweets and junk food. He was anointed with oil while a few of us lads laid hands on him. I prayed that Laurie would find comfort in Christ – not the Blue Ribands in the common room biscuit tin. And that his late-night snaffles would turn into late-night prayers.

Friday 28 January

I found one of the more theologically opinionated ordinands quietly sulking in a darkened corner of the common room before breakfast. He was lamenting after receiving another low mark in his systematics essay and trying to make sense of the red pen scrawled over his paper. This guy reads the likes of St Augustine for fun. But he's all strong opinions and no analysis. He doesn't have the intellectual or theological wriggle room to frame a proper argument or tickle our markers in the right places. He looked surprised and disappointed with my high mark. 'How did you manage that?' he asked me. He emphasized the 'you' a bit too much. I shared my essay-writing secrets but I could tell he wasn't listening.

I'm such a Pharisee at times. I grinned with smug satisfaction that someone on Bible reading duty had slept in for Morning Prayer. There was an empty chair beside Rob Lee as he led. Someone was in for it, I mused (a bit too gleefully). About ten minutes in, it dawned on me that I hadn't checked the rota for a while. I looked afterwards. It was my turn. I did the honourable thing and blamed Rob for not letting me know.

After last week's incendiary pioneer ministry seminar, our tutor reminded us that we were actually Christians so it would be good for us to stop shouting at each other. He put it far more sensitively than that. As a result, the session was far more sedate and pleasant but a bit dull. I think a good verbal tear-up is really healthy from time to time. It's good for the soul. It's what we're here for. We're signing up for a lifetime of being nice and reasonable and holding all sides of the argument in steady tension when we start in our parishes. I want to put that off until the last possible moment and express how I really feel now – proudly and loudly and at times unreasonably.

Saturday 29 January

I looked after the babies all night at Mum's so Anna could sleep. It gave me a window into her world right now. Heidi was awake from 9 p.m. to 7 a.m. I took comfort from the fact that every hour that passed was another hour that Anna was resting.

Ian has treated me to a ticket to see Liam Gallagher's new band Beady Eye in Liverpool. He's back in my good books. Ian knows what being within spitting distance of Liam means to me. I've been asked if I'll be interviewed by Radio 4 about faith and doubt. I reluctantly agreed. Radio 4 is a bit too high brow for me. I'm more Galaxy FM.

I did something unbelievably stupid tonight. I sent Stuart a very snotty, overly aggressive email to complain about the 58 per cent mark he gave me in my essay. Never send an email when you're angry. Definitely never send one when you're absolutely fuming. I felt the mark was too low and his feedback comments patronizing. It pushed all my insecurity buttons. Anna had pleaded with me not to send the email. I didn't listen. Now I'm regretting it.

Monday 31 January

To say Stuart hasn't taken my email very well is an understatement. He has demanded to see me as soon as possible. I managed to dodge him all day. It wouldn't be helpful right now. I'm still too angry. Feeling rejection in this way takes me into the danger zone where I don't know what I'm capable of saying.

A letter was read out at our full Cranmer common room committee meeting on behalf of Aidan. In his unofficial capacity as student spokesman, he has moved on from trying to singlehandedly raise the standards of teaching in our lectures. Now he's seeking to improve the quality and quantity of our community prayer life. The letter said that ordinands had been skipping prayer meetings. It stressed how detrimental this was to us as individuals and the Cranmer community as a whole. Endless scriptures were quoted. Aidan isn't wrong (we do need to pray more). I know he would have written the letter in good faith and with integrity. But it was so patronizing. I wrote the minutes in such a way as to make Paul and me howl with laughter. Sometimes it's all you can do in this place.

Tuesday 1 February

Stuart finally cornered me about 'emailgate'. As expected, he gave me both barrels. It has brought to the surface some anger and rejection issues that I thought were long since dealt with. I don't want to overdramatize it (not easy for me), but this felt like a significant moment for me as a man, a future priest and follower of Christ. I'd clearly wounded Stuart. He's undeniably godly and full of integrity. It's funny how someone as laid back as Stuart can suddenly turn into a dead-eyed ninja when they need to.

He darted straight out of Morning Prayer and collared me. It was a long walk to his office. It felt like the time at secondary school when Miss Williamson took me to see the head after I was caught hitting Duncan Batchelor in the nose with my pencil case. Stuart shook with anger as he told me how out of order it was to send that email to a 'brother in Christ'. I stupidly tried to defend it at first. I asked if he thought he was being 'a bit sensitive'. That didn't go down well. I capitulated. I knew I was wrong. There was no mitigation. I apologized unreservedly and asked for forgiveness. Then we prayed.

During the Peace at college Communion tonight Stuart and I sought each other out for a man hug. We spoke wonderful words of reconciliation to each other in that moment. And I thought the Peace was just that awkward bit of the service that makes newcomers, introverts and those paranoid about whether to hug or handshake squirm. Stuart is a class act. I'm so grateful he's my tutor. We will move on.

Wednesday 2 February

Rhys Thomas has agreed to run a marathon with me before we leave Cranmer. I wanted to do something in memory of Aunty Lynne and raise a few quid for cancer research. We're calling our appeal 'Running for Aunty Lynne'.

Saturday 5 February

'Edifying' is my new favourite word. I'm using it all the time in open conversation.

Monday 7 February

I attended my first St John's College formal dinner tonight with Paul. We wore borrowed suits and academic gowns to blend in with the undergrads. It was like being in a period drama. It could have been 1927. All I needed was a monocle and a silver cigarette case. I sat with the Junior Common Room President and a guy reading science and maths. They talked about scientists like I talk about footy players. I wondered if there was a Panini sticker album equivalent when they were kids?

They regaled me with stories about some of the great unsolved maths theorems. One of them is called the Riemann hypothesis. There's still a £1 million prize for anyone who can solve it. The lads discussed their subject with such passion and wide-eyed wonder. It was infectious. Maths and science, infectious. Wow. I'm either becoming unbelievably dull or they were extraordinarily interesting. Probably the latter.

Tuesday 8 February

Reading Leviticus 24.10–23 has unsettled me. No matter how I interpret it, I still can't seem to equate the God we find there with the God of Jesus Christ. Verses 13 and 14 are a good example: 'The Lord said to Moses: "Take the blasphemer outside the camp; and let all who were within hearing lay their hands on his head, and then let the whole congregation stone him."' That's just what they did as verse 23 documents: 'Moses spoke thus to the people of Israel; and they took the blasphemer outside the camp, and stoned him to death. The people of Israel did as the Lord had commanded Moses.' I tried to imagine Jesus making that decision. He wouldn't, would he? I shared my disorientation with the Morning Glory boys. They were unusually quiet. Even Aidan.

Wednesday 9 February

I've received a lovely email from Anna. She wanted to tell me how happy and content she is. It makes me happy to know that she's happy. There's a wonderful serenity about her now.

Harry and I spent our placement quiet day at St Antony's Priory. Not all of it was quiet, mind you. Far from it. It was my kind of retreat day, though. There were periods of silence and prayer, but also plenty of reading, dreaming and laughter. We opened up about the reality of married life and how Anna and Ruth fit into our calling to become reverends. They're not typical vicars' wives. They don't know how to make quiche for a start. They're shy, too. They don't want to spend their lives on a tea rota. This could be a frustration to us but it shouldn't be. We each wrote them a letter that we'll probably never send. They lay out our fears, frustrations and failures. Harry is so annoyingly creative. During one of our quiet spells, he composed a modern-day hymn based on Psalm 30.

The day ended with cries of laughter as we discovered that our day's fasting had given us terrible breath. Harry's tongue was banana-coloured.

Thursday 10 February

Aidan and I had a heart to heart after Night Prayer. We've decided that our Lenten discipline will be to make every effort not to argue, bicker or provoke. We want to find common ground. He later tweeted: 'I love Matt Woodcock. He annoys me but I think we believe the same thing – that we want people to know Jesus Christ.' At last, something we agree on.

Friday 11 February

The babies were asleep when I got back to York. Anna gave me the look. It was on. I literally sprinted up to the bedroom to put on my birthday suit. A few glasses of Prosecco later and the rest is history. It was probably still too early for Anna. 'It's like getting back on a bike,' I told her. 'We're going to have to get a lot of practice.' Heidi then woke up and all hell broke loose.

Tuesday 15 February

For the good of his craft and his future in theological academia, I wish I'd had the guts to gently tell our new student lecturer how unhelpfully dull and uninspiring his session was today. He seems like a lovely guy, but if he doesn't learn now he'll go on teaching like this. The poor guy has no comprehension that the mysteries of Isaiah will not be unlocked by him blandly jawing at us for two hours. We need space to discuss, debate and wrestle. I want to learn how this stuff relates to people's real lives, otherwise what's the point of it? Someone needs to tell him. Sensitively. So it can't be me.

In my tutorial with Stuart, he pinpointed some key ministerial skills I still need to work on. They include listening, learning when to shut up and patience. I may need more time.

Cringe moments continue to plague me. A leading evangelical on the preaching circuit spoke at our college Communion tonight. A few of us were loudly and ungenerously pulling apart his sermon in the corridor afterwards. I was particularly harsh. Then a toilet flushed and the guy stepped into the corridor. He must have heard the whole thing. I felt awkward, wretched and feeble. I've got to start being a better human being. All the major lessons I'm learning at Cranmer are happening outside the lecture hall.

Friday 18 February

Rhys and I got up at 5.30 a.m. to run 13 miles. It took us 1 hour 58 minutes. We're taking the opportunity to pray for people as we run round. It takes our mind off the pain. The hills are brutal. Every mile counts as we prepare for the Druridge Bay Marathon on 15 May. There's no greater time to run than as the dawn breaks. Except when you're hungover. Then it's hideous.

My pioneer ministry group went on an outing today to a struggling former mining community called Sacriston. I'd have preferred Alton Towers, to be honest. In pairs, the brief was to walk, observe, reflect and pray. It's a depressing place. The Anglican church looked so unloved and unwelcoming. The notice board outside annoyed me. The minister's name was followed by a list of academic awards and letters, filling an entire line. How to put distance between you and the people before even meeting them. The walk was a stimulating time for Harry and me. If we're honest, most of us in the group would want to be placed anywhere but here. That's usually when God starts to smile. Harry had bogies hanging out of his nose all day. It was too funny to point them out to him.

Saturday 19 February

Watching *The Blind Side* broke me tonight. I can't cope with the scene where the Sandra Bullock character takes in Big Mike. I want to be more like that. Christ calls us to be more like that.

Wednesday 23 February

Preparing my sermon on Ephesians 5, I remembered a great story about Christian activist Tony Campolo. He'd grown increasingly disturbed about the number of prostitutes working near his church. One night he decided to act. Tony gathered together about six of the women and paid for their time for a whole evening. They ate pizzas, watched films and put the world to rights. The next day Tony addressed his church and said: 'I had a brilliant time with six prostitutes last night!'

I was inspired to write a song tonight after finishing reading *Schindler's Ark*. I somehow wanted to articulate my feelings about the evil of the camp commandant Amon Göth. I likened his unspeakable horrors to one of Francis Bacon's paintings. Few artists depict the blackness of the human soul like him. My song failed on every level. Rhyming 'evil glint' with 'heart like a Bacon print' was up there with the worst of my sixth-form poetry.

Saturday 26 February

I've completed my 'Thought for the Day' to read out to our preaching class next week. Dad told me not to change a word of it. High praise indeed. Writing for radio is different to what I'm used to. Full stops and commas are crucial in conveying a sense of surprise, power and meaning to a sentence. Alistair Cooke is the benchmark.

I read another one of those 'Ouch' verses during my morning Bible study. Numbers 15.35 says: 'Then the Lord said to Moses, "This man must die. The whole assembly must stone him outside the camp."' The man's crime? Gathering wood on the Sabbath day. Jesus would not have ordered that man's death. Would he?

Sunday 27 February

I'm struck this week by how blessed I am. How abundantly I live. In no particular order, there's the food, roof, children, wife, family, friends, health and God. I need to get better at sharing it.

Monday 28 February

I'm fuming that Paul Bromley has trounced me in the leadership essay. He got 68 to my 63. That's unheard of. I begrudgingly bought him a bag of Maltesers to congratulate his win. My assessors said I'd put too much emphasis on the effectiveness of my own leadership rather than on the leaders around me. One of the markers clearly thinks I'm the next David Koresh or something. He wrote: 'There could be a dangerous vanity about your future ministry.' Charismatic leaders with a personality are not encouraged in the Church of England. So I've decided to pray and fast every lunchtime over Lent. Hopefully it will help me be less dangerously vain.

Tuesday 1 March

Our student lecturer has soared in my estimations. Not only did he fail to turn up to give today's seminar – but he was refreshingly honest enough to email us an apology and tell us why. He said he'd slept in. No excuses, no wriggling, no rubbish. Just an honest comment that he'd overslept. Brilliant. What a class act. I emailed him back: 'Don't worry, buddy – it happens to the best of us!' People's raw honesty makes me really happy.

Wednesday 2 March

My 'Thought for the Day' was greeted with silence by the preaching class. Writing the script has taken an emotional toll. Auschwitz is one of those subjects where a colourful imagination can have consequences to the soul. It's no wonder that so many of the great chroniclers of war and conflict were mad drunks. I think it's worth recording my piece in full:

In two days' time I will be at the place where 1.1 million people were murdered. Such was the evil and depravity of Auschwitz, some say that it is both physically and spiritually dead. The wildlife keep away. The birds don't sing. That it is permanently cold and dark. Some are also adamant that God does not exist there. That he never has. That he never could have done. As someone on the verge of ordination to the priesthood, I want to go and find out for myself. To say I am apprehensive is an understatement.

In preparation, I have recently immersed myself in Auschwitz literature. Much of it is nightmarish, as you would expect. A particular photograph has haunted me. It depicts two lines of people beside the camp's railway track. Men in one line, women and children in the other. They are waiting to be selected, either for work or death. There is a Jewish woman frantically looking over at the male line, presumably at her husband. She is holding a baby who is nuzzling against her cheek, oblivious to the horror all around. Oblivious to the imminence of murder. As a new father of twelve weeks this image has been particularly hard to deal with or even comprehend.

I sat with a colleague in a quiet chapel to mark Holocaust Memorial Day recently. We tried to articulate words of prayer. Words of grace came out of my mouth, but, if I'm honest, thoughts of hate and contempt for those SS guards were not far away. And yet I've also been given cause to hope. Primo Levi's evocative memoir of his Auschwitz experience, If This Is a Man, *tells of an encounter with a camp inmate he barely knew called Lorenzo. Through an act of inexplicable, extreme kindness by this man, Levi is reawakened and revitalized. 'I believe that it was really due to Lorenzo that I am alive today,' he writes. 'And not so much for his material aid, as for his having constantly reminded me by his presence, by his natural and plain manner of being good, that there still existed a just world outside our own. Something and someone still pure and whole, not corrupt, not savage, extraneous to hatred and terror, something difficult to define, a remote possibility of good for which it was worth surviving.'*

So I hope when walking among the long-faded footsteps of those 1.1 million victims, that I discover the truth in the words of the Apostle John. That 'light shines in the darkness and the darkness did not overcome it'. My faith depends on it.

Friday 4 March

We've done the likes of Madrid, Barcelona, San Francisco, Rome, Ghent, Prague, Paris and Antwerp. When money was tight we did Lincoln. This weekend it's Kraków. My yearly adventures with Dad are the glue that keeps us together. They make our relationship make sense. I realize now that we cram a year's worth of love, pain, spirituality and laughter into four days. We need this. He may have been a rubbish father in the conventional sense, but there is still no human being I find more illuminating or interesting than him. For these four days a year, anyway. We gathered outside The Old Grey Mare at 4.15 a.m. to drive to John Lennon Airport. Aside from an old couple and us, our Easyjet flight was packed with three noisy stag dos. It was mayhem. A gang of middle-aged Scousers were the most entertaining group. They seemed to relish being let off the leash. Their stag – 'Stan' – was made to suffer. They plied him with spirits, insults and threats about what was in store for him in Kraków's bars and brothels. He couldn't stand up by the time we landed. Lord, have mercy on Stan.

Kraków is like something from a John le Carré spy novel. It's cold, misty and full of atmosphere. With a full day to devour, we sought to dodge the stags and go in search of the real Kraków. Inevitably that led us to a bar. It looked out onto the old town's main square. The sun poured onto our faces, taking the edge off the cold nip. On these trips, we instinctively go in search of the ultimate interlude. This was one.

Dad put the square in its historical context. He demands that I use my imagination. He kept reminding me that the square is where Oskar Schindler and the Nazis would have walked. He won't rest until I can see what he's seeing. He is the best kind of tour guide. But his bladder is shot. Minutes after leaving the square to explore, Dad was sprinting to find somewhere to pee. He dived into what looked like a Frankie and Benny's-style restaurant called Pod Wawelem.

It was a wonderful fluke. The next few hours were so full of joy, depth and ridiculously large beers that I thought my heart would explode. Everything about Pod Wawelem is on an industrial scale. Its unique selling point is that they will stuff you so full of deliciously rustic food that you will probably be physically sick. They've even made provisions for such an eventuality. The toilets have a dedicated vomit section. They want patrons to make room to keep gorging. Madness! We laughed hard at the thought of it. Tears ran down Dad's face. After some complimentary cherry vodka shots, we staggered out to explore the Jewish quarter. Strong coffee just about averted the infamous 'Kraków hangover'. We didn't verbalize it, but our visit to Auschwitz tomorrow loomed heavy on our minds.

Saturday 5 March

Part of me will never be quite the same after experiencing Auschwitz-Birkenau. The horror of what happened there will always be with me now. I write this still unable to take it in, to properly comprehend, to believe that it could be true. I walked where 1.5 million people were murdered just because they were Jewish, gypsy, disabled, left wing, gay or just a bit different. Wandering in and out of the sleeping quarters, gas chambers, prison cells, station platform and places of execution was the most numbing experience of my life. Every school pupil should be made to come here. Words of prayer were difficult to come by. God was present, though. I'm sure of it. There was light even in this place of terrible darkness. Maybe the darkest place in the history of the world.

Accounts of goodness and hope peppered the evil, like the faintest smattering of stars on the blackest night. There's too much to take in. It's interesting what becomes embedded. For me, it was a photo of a female survivor taken on the day the camp was liberated. It was the face of a 50-year-old woman. She was actually

14. Her haunted, hunted eyes had seen things no human being ever should. Then there was the swimming pool where the commandant's children played and swam. It was a wall's width from the gas chamber and ovens. Screams of childish pleasure side by side with screams of death. I wish I hadn't noticed the photographs of hundreds of babies of Esther and Heidi's age piled up in a mass grave. I noticed a suitcase belonging to a Jewish girl called Anna.

I was also struck by the story of the Sonderkommando who tried to kill himself by walking into a gas chamber with a group of his fellow Jews. They pushed him back out with the challenge, 'go and bear witness'. The memorial at Birkenau summed it up best:

Forever let this place be a cry of despair and a warning to humanity, where the Nazis murdered about 1.5 million men, women and children, mainly Jews, from various countries of Europe. Auschwitz-Birkenau 1940–1945.

Like the Sonderkommando, anyone who has visited this place must bear witness. Dad said he couldn't fathom how so many German soldiers could have been complicit in the mass murder. And so many ordinary German citizens stood by and let it happen. Would we have been any different in England?

We needed a drink when we got back to Kraków. It was important to unpack how we felt. Inevitably, the subject of Jesus Christ came up. It always does with Dad. He weeps at the very mention of his name. I asked him: 'How can you know so much about Jesus and believe what he said, but not actually follow him?' He replied: 'How do you know I don't?' I nearly choked on my beer. He's never said that before. We stopped off at a cellar bar for coffee near the hotel. On a day of extreme emotions, it was lovely to descend into inane conversation. We tried to name the actors who played *The Magnificent Seven*. Dad managed six of them.

I couldn't bear not knowing the seventh. I texted Uncle Mike to find out. It was Brad Dexter.

Sunday 6 March

A bitterly cold, subdued day. We were still emotionally reeling. Dad has aged significantly. He has developed that condition where a blob of snot hangs precariously from the end of his nose. He doesn't realize it until you point it out. He's getting irritated that I keep pointing it out.

We explored the castle and the cathedral where John Paul II was based as Archbishop before he became Pope. We sat in on the 10 a.m. service. I couldn't understand a word. It made me think of visitors who experience the same thing in our churches back home. We so often talk in a foreign language, even though we're speaking English.

Monday 7 March

I've never seen so many hungover blokes in my life than at Kraków's airport departure lounge. We sat near a lively group who looked like they hadn't slept for four days. They bragged about beer, dancing and brothel conquests. One of the biggest lessons we've learnt on this trip is not to judge. We sniffily dismissed Stan and his middle-aged stag-do gang on the first day. On the flight over we presumed they were only in Poland for the beer and prostitutes. I even said to Dad: '*They* won't be going to Auschwitz.' I was wrong. They were on the same tour as us. Stan's gang. Silent and numb like the rest of us. Tears rolling down their faces.

How appropriate that I'm reading Henri Nouwen's reflections on Rembrandt's painting *The Return of the Prodigal Son*. His thoughts on the prodigal's older brother spoke to me deeply. Nouwen writes: 'Time and again I discover within me that murmuring, whining, grumbling, lamenting and griping that go on and on even against my will … condemnation of others and self-condemnation, self-righteousness and self-rejection keep reinforcing each other in an ever more vicious way.' There's a bit of the older brother in all of us.

The welcome was colder than Kraków when I arrived home. Mum, Amy and Anna were hostile. They weren't happy with me being away. There's a feeling that I could be doing more to help Anna. They have a point but I hope they see the importance of this trip in time. I dread to think what reception Stan got from his fiancée. His eyebrows will take some growing back.

Tuesday 8 March

Lent fever has gripped Cranmer. The place is abuzz with talk about what people are giving up or taking up. Some of us are so self-righteous. We're essentially trying to out-penance each other. The fasts are getting longer, the personal sacrifices more extreme. I usually talk a good Lent. I announced shamelessly loudly in the common room that I was fasting my mid-week lunches and replacing them with meditative prayer. I'm determined to stick to it. I'm not being outdone by Aidan this year. Jesus had something to say about religious people like us. It wasn't complimentary.

Wednesday 9 March

I completed my first Lenten lunch fast today. I could have murdered a plate of chips. It's a good discipline for me though. I lay on my bed holding a comfort cross, imagining myself with Jesus again in the back of that rickety cart. My mind wandered as my tummy rumbled.

We experienced a powerful Anglo-Catholic-style service in the chapel tonight. I can't work out whether David keeps falling asleep during the worship or if he's praying. I'd forgive him the occasional catnap. He's putting the hours in as Cranmer's interim boss.

I embarrassed myself in the college bar afterwards. One of the senior lecturers was having a quiet pint as I held court in the corner. He got up to leave and I shouted after him: 'I'll be up in ten minutes, darling.' No one laughed. He said he didn't hear me so I had to repeat it. It was even less funny second time round. He rolled his eyes wearily and went to bed. Why would I say that?! Cringe.

Thursday 10 March

The closer I get to ordination the more I seem to be unravelling. I stormed out of our Morning Glory prayer meeting after another disagreement with Aidan. I know he's struggling but his constant negativity and critiquing of the Church sent me over the edge. I shouted at him that his attitude was destructive and unhelpful to those of us becoming revs in just a few months' time. I slammed the door behind me a bit too dramatically. We all kissed and made up over breakfast. The boys were forgiving. They understood.

Friday 11 March

Long-distance running and fasting is a terrible combination. Rhys and I were up at 5.30 a.m. for a 13-miler. I had a funny turn after 8 miles. I ate loads of pasta last night but clearly my body was missing those lunches. We're aiming for a sub-4-hour marathon.

Aidan seems to be right on the verge of a meltdown. He had a face like thunder in lectures today. I'm worried about him. For all our issues I love the guy. I want good things for him.

Saturday 12 March

I guess it happens to most husbands when children arrive. But it dawned on me how marginalized I've become. Anna's primary focus is the girls. I know it has to be that way but I am a selfish Neanderthal. It's taking some adjusting to. All dads go through this, I'm sure. It doesn't help that I'm in Durham all week, but what else can I do? Mum went on the offensive when I popped round. She questioned my dad skills and the level of support I give to Anna. I huffed and puffed. The truth hurts. I need to do better.

Sunday 13 March

Radio 4 broadcast the faith and doubt feature this afternoon. The stellar contributors included Rowan Williams, one of the country's leading Christian scientists – and me. My point was that doubt is part of being a Christian. I told the interviewer that I'm interested in leading a church that's fuzzy-edged enough to allow honest and open discussion about life's real doubts, joys and struggles. Rowan said basically the same thing – only far more quietly and lucidly.

Wednesday 16 March

Discipleship group worship was a joy this morning. Stephen led a meditation based on something monks use called *Lectio Divina* (literally, 'holy reading'). It was so simple. There were no pebbles to suck, flowing streams to listen to or candles to stare at. It was just Stephen reading from the Bible. He has a gift. He sounds like Alec Guinness in *Star Wars*.

I hate coming across as weak or lily-livered, but I felt compelled to see our college warden David about my home situation. It was in light of the latest college missive instructing us that we were all expected at a special Monday morning Communion to celebrate the life of Thomas Cranmer. I explained that Anna was at breaking point. She'd had enough of feeling like a single parent. I said that the guilt of being away so much was doing my head in. 'I like Thomas Cranmer, David,' I said, 'but I'm not willing to get divorced over the guy.' He was so understanding and pastoral. He reassured me that I had 'a blank cheque' to come and go as I pleased. We agreed that I would now work from home on Mondays.

Thursday 17 March

In New Testament we debated the tricky subject of what actually *happens* to the bread and wine during the Eucharist. Do the elements become the actual, physical body and blood of Jesus Christ? Or is it more symbolic? A range of views were offered. I agreed with our lecturer. Something powerful is happening in that moment, but God is not as concerned as we are about it as long as he receives the honour and the glory.

Paul Bromley persuaded me to hit the town tonight. I didn't put up much of a fight. It was glorious. We went to the college bar for 'one drink'. It was heaving with students in fancy dress for St Patrick's Day. We mingled with male rugby players dressed as scantily clad netball players and female netball players dressed as rugby players in the shortest of shorts. Paul had a permanent smile on his face. We discussed how realistic it was to truly be ourselves as priests. God has called us as we are, we know that. But it will be a struggle not to conform to the likeness of so many of the vicars we know. Then again, having this conversation in a packed, deafening bar full of conga-ing party people perhaps answered our own question.

We found Thapelo looking lost on the way out. We persuaded him to join us for a pint. He calls it 'imbibing'. He joined in our discussions about the priesthood. Thapelo has a very 'high' view of it. He actually believes that priests have 'special powers'. That the ordained are somehow on a higher spiritual plain. I disagreed. Surely Christ calls us to be smelly-feet-washers, not heaven-gazing holy Joes? That's the deal. Paul and I ended up nightclubbing in Osbournes. We sang our hearts out to cheesy pop. We felt 19 again wobbling back to our college digs clutching Subway's Footlongs. We bumped into the St John's College student president arm in arm with a young lady. He looked wonderfully sheepish. I challenged him to a sprint race back to college. He won convincingly. I think I've pulled a tendon. This was one of the great Cranmer nights. That 'one quiet drink' has a lot to answer for.

Friday 18 March

Archbishop Sentamu came to Cranmer today to encourage and inspire us. We had a good catch-up afterwards. I've missed working with him at Bishopthorpe. He has been such an influence on my journey. I'm not sure I would have got to this point without his encouragement. He had such faith that we would have children in some of our darkest days of doubt and despair. I'll never forget him praying for Anna in his chapel before I left for Durham. He prayed like he expected God to bless us with kids. There's a presence about Sentamu that compels me to keep believing and following. His message today was simple and direct: follow Christ's example. Live out his calling and go and make disciples. I can live with that.

Sunday 20 March

The vicar who made it possible for our daughters to be born held them for the first time at their baptism today. His gesture to pay for the IVF treatment – twice – was a game-changer for us. We've never experienced such Christ-like generosity and radical hopefulness. Esther and Heidi would simply not exist without him. He prayed a blessing over the girls as he cradled them in his arms. He said that helping us was 'one of the best things' he'd ever done in his life. St Paul's made everything really special for the baptism. Balloons were hung everywhere. Someone had made delicious cakes. The service itself was wonderful chaos. Just how we like it. The curate, Mike, interviewed me. I shared what this day meant to us in light of those bleak childless years. It was Mike's first baptism as a new curate. I didn't let that pass. 'On a scale of one to ten, Mike, how nervous are you about dropping our beautiful, precious babies?!' I asked.

Thursday 24 March

I've just burst into the senior common room to chastise three drunken students for being too loud. It is late. One of them was being sick into a bin. His friend was close to tears as he spluttered an apology. It turns out he's going to be president of the Christian Union next year. No wonder he was so sheepish. When did I start telling people off for a bit of drunken noise? It's a slippery slope. How long will it be before I'm thinking that sandals and socks are an acceptable combination or gardening a worthwhile pastime on my day off?

Friday 25 March

It's all getting very real now. Ordination looms. I don't feel ready. I'm scared. We've come away to a secluded retreat house for the Cranmer leavers' weekend. It's a silent retreat. Instinctively I wanted to rebel. My natural instinct is to be heard. To say something. Being silent for three days seems unrealistic when you're sharing a room with Paul Bromley. His hairy bulk demands words. We'd originally planned to stuff the rules and sneak off to the pub after Compline. But something stopped us. Or someone. For all our blokey bluster, we know how important this could be. So we've made a pact to honour the silence. We won't say a word.

I'm determined to take the opportunity to really listen to God. It's something I don't do enough of. I feel strongly that he's got business to do with me. Things he wants to tell me. So, my weekend retreat policy is this: mouth shut, eyes closed, heart open.

I feel guilty about leaving Anna and the girls all weekend but what could I do? She texted to say how she'd love some silence right now. Ouch. I'm in awe of Anna. Since the birth, she is far more self-conscious about her body. She's worried that I won't desire her in the same way because she's droopier, saggier and scarred. I actually marvel at her body in a fresh way. Her milk-filled breasts are wonderful. Her stretch marks are a thing of beauty. They're like battle scars – symbols of her courage, patience and endurance.

These thoughts aren't healthy for me right now. I'm writing this from a tiny room in a bed next to Paul. He's snoring like a pregnant sow. And I can't even shout and swear at him to shut up because of my vow of silence. How annoying.

Saturday 26 March

The only words I've spoken all day have been to God. That's a world first. The love of Christ broke me. The reality of it flooded my heart afresh. I know how super-spiritual that sounds. It's the kind of sentence that if someone else said it my eyes would roll. But stuff happened between me and God today. Big stuff.

Lying on the bed after breakfast, I was filled with remorse for living my own way too often. I wept as I asked for forgiveness. It felt liberating and exciting. I felt whole again. It dawned on me how all-consuming and frenetic my life has become. It's no wonder I struggle to hear God sometimes. I don't listen.

My head was pounding when I woke up. I'd planned to use the quiet to get busy with sermon-writing and this and that. The headache forced me to lie down and do nothing except listen to God. That's when things started to stir within my deepest, dustiest places.

Things got even more interesting by late afternoon. I had a St Cuthbert-type moment during a walk in the grounds. It's not easy to articulate in words. Anyone reading this will think I've gone nuts. I stood on some raised ground overlooking a wood. Suddenly I became unmistakably aware of God's presence in everything I saw, heard and felt. Nature seemed to come alive. I could see his hand at work in the myriad colours of the trees, and in the noise of the flowing stream. The rich abundance of the wood overwhelmed me. It was like my soul was singing a psalm of praise.

It's important for me to record this because I will deny to myself that it ever happened over time. This was a gift. God made absolute sense. Seldom has he felt so close or Jesus so real. I walked into the heart of the wood and shouted out to God all my thanks, hopes and fears. He heard me. I hope no one else did. That would have been well embarrassing.

Sunday 27 March

After our final Eucharist, I couldn't get away fast enough. I knew I would struggle to do a quick transition from silent to sociable. I needed to come down gently. The silence has been a nightmare for some of the group. One guy demonstrated how you can still be loud in non-verbal ways, though – burping, farting, shuffling, sighing, texting and tweeting. We heard him all right.

Before breakfast, I returned to my special spot to watch the sun rise over the fir trees. The morning dew sparkled like tinsel on the grass. I caught sight of Joel Wood wandering around like John the Baptist. The Psalms come alive on mornings like this. In the silence of this weekend, God's voice has been deafening.

Sunday 3 April

This was the day Anna always dreaded. A day to think about the flowers she'd never get, and card that would never be made for her. Not any more. I brought her crumpets in bed. She had the pleasure of opening two Mother's Day cards. The girls couldn't be more different right now. Esther is grumpy and hostile. Heidi is a gurgling smiler. Today was one of those rare occasions when Anna unfurled her heart to let me see inside. She wrote me this card: 'I know it has turned into a commercial racket but I always felt sad in years gone by, wondering if I would ever have children to collect flowers for me at church – and now look! Two beautiful daughters! What a blessing! Thank you, God!'

Excruciating 'cringe' moments seem to be happening to me on a daily basis. I'd noticed our neighbour, Bill, washing his car yesterday. As I drove past, I wound down my window and jokingly said: 'Will you run a wet cloth over mine when you're finished please, Bill?' As I pulled out of the drive tonight he ran over all excited. 'So what do you think?' he asked. It was only then I noticed that he'd actually given my car a full clean and polish. What a special guy, but how awfully embarrassing. One beautiful day I will learn to keep my mouth shut.

Monday 4 April

In preparation for today's conflict resolution class we had to fill out a questionnaire. It asked how we handled people in a range of scenarios. We got a total score based on our answers. My score of 40 was something of an anomaly, apparently. A worrying extreme. The assessors took me to one side for 'a quiet word'. According to their analysis, scoring a 40 means I could achieve great things in my future church ministry. The downside is that there's a good chance I could be a magnet for conflict. The feedback sheet reported that someone in my category, 'Readily accepts difficult challenges'. We are people of 'high energy'. We 'quickly win the confidence of others'. We are a 'source of ideas, possibilities. Forward looking, optimistic. Inspire higher level of performance from others.' The downsides are that we can often 'innovate to avoid boredom' and 'other people's standard performances become sub-standard by comparison'. Most worryingly of all, we have a tendency to 'manipulate and abuse others' loyalty and integrity'. So, in summary, I'll be a force for positive change in the Church of England, but could end up defrocked by my second year.

We had a leaving presentation for Thapelo this afternoon. He cried his eyes out. It's amazing to think that he'll be doing ministry on horseback when he returns to his mountainous parish in Lesotho. I'll miss the little guy.

Wednesday 6 April

Anna's paranoia about the girls' health has intensified. She's now concerned that Esther might be autistic because she doesn't do eye contact. The health visitor seemed unconcerned. Anna is now banned from surfing the mummy internet sites.

Friday 8 April

I got a helpful insight into how others see me today. Mike – one of the more aloof lads at college – texted this: 'I had my hair cut in Durham today by a lovely blonde lass. She told me that she'd recently had this excitable Yorkshireman in the chair who had been going mad over the prospect of a weekend of silence! "I get all the nutters," she said. Any idea who she was talking about?!' How funny. I remember that conversation. I need to calm down a bit.

Saturday 9 April

Evangelicals are going into meltdown over a new book by the super-cool US pastor Rob Bell. The guy is taking a lot of stick for his views in *Love Wins*. It takes a fresh look at what happens when we die. I found myself getting involved and berating the guy's theology without having read the thing. That's never good (or 'cool', as he would say). So I found Bell's email online and wrote him an apology. Among other things, it said: 'As a future church leader I should have known better.' I should. Saying sorry always feels good.

I needed more forgiveness after coming back from my marathon practice run this evening. Pounding across Tadcaster Road with my headphones on, a car nearly hit me. It didn't miss by much. The fist-waving driver did that really annoying thing of holding his hand down on the horn. I lost it. Shouting expletives at him, I chased after his Audi as it sped away. With the benefit of hindsight I'm trying to picture how that looked to the general public. Not great. I felt utterly ridiculous once I'd calmed down. I could see the headline: 'Maniac rookie rev arrested for run rage'. I've got to keep reminding myself that I'm only a few months away from being ordained.

Sunday 10 April

I'm not doing very well as a dad. Going in to check on the twins this morning, I discovered a massive bumblebee crawling over Esther's tummy. I panicked and ran to get Anna. How pathetic. So far, out of 10, I'd give my fathering skills a low 4.

Tuesday 12 April

I think I'm having a pre-rev-life crisis. I crowd-surfed for the first time while watching Liam Gallagher's band Beady Eye with Ian in Liverpool tonight. It was one of the most euphoric experiences of my life. We positioned ourselves near the back of the venue to begin with for Ian's sake. He's more of a reserved head-bobber at gigs. But as soon as Liam strutted onto the stage I couldn't contain myself. Suddenly the man I've tried to mimic in front of countless mirrors since my late teens was stood before me. I surged into the middle of a group of Liam diehards at the front. They were pretty ferocious, menacing and drunk. But during these songs they were brothers, fellow worshippers at the church of St Liam.

During the final song I became overwhelmed in the sweaty rapture of the moment. I noticed a few lads being hoisted up and carried to the front by the crowd. The shaven-headed scouser next to me noticed my face peak with interest at the possibility of such an experience. Before I knew it, he'd lifted me above his head. Raised hands took my weight and began to surf me around. I screamed and writhed with delight. Time was suspended as I looked upon the sea of sweaty faces. It was a few seconds of ecstasy. I'm sure Liam and I shared *a moment*. He seemed to give me a nod of respect. Or was it a signal to security that a nutter was being surfed his way?

My euphoria was short-lived. I was suddenly dumped headfirst into the security pit by the merciless front row. My neck felt like it teetered on the edge of a break. On nights like this every part of me wants to resist becoming a reverend. I feel like I'm getting ready for a life in a cage where my every move will be scrutinized and judged. I want to live freely and spontaneously. And irresponsibly at times. I want to be where real people are and real life is happening. Is that possible with a dog collar on?

Wednesday 13 April

Jo came round to see us tonight before going back to Doha. It was heart-breaking. She is utterly grief-stricken. Life has become something for her to endure since Aunty Lynne died. My words of comfort sounded hollow and ineffectual. What could I say? To see someone I love in so much pain and not being able to fix it is intensely frustrating.

I thought back to our early years together as cousins, confidantes and kindred spirits. She was the closest person to me for the first 15 years of my life. Through toddlers, nursery, primary and secondary school we did *everything* together. I did everything she said. Her opinion, her approval, was crucial. Jo actually negotiated and arranged my first kiss. There weren't many weekends when I wasn't sleeping on her floor trying not to wake Uncle Ally with our belly laughs. When Jo dipped her toe in the waters of faith, I soon dived in. But now here she was in our front room, grieving, broken and numb. I could do nothing about it. Before leaving, Jo said to me: 'I know you've got a strong faith, Matt, but I don't believe any of it any more. Life is just too cruel.'

Thursday 14 April

I continue to have major doubts about my calling. It would help if I actually liked going to church. I can't sleep for worrying about that dog collar going round my neck. Will it drive the passion out of me? Will it change who I am? I couldn't live life as some kind of holy fraud. My attitude towards the traditional way of doing church still worries me. I can't ever imagine a Sunday when I won't find some element of it dull or joyless. Is that normal? Am I signing up to a life of encouraging people to come into a cold, decaying, alien building that is living on its history but dying in its reality?

And yet. God loves his Church. He sees possibilities and opportunities everywhere. Deep down I know he calls me to do the same. It's terrifying (but also quite comical) that he wants me to help breathe new life into it. Starting at Holy Trinity in July.

Tuesday 19 April

Our 21-mile training run was full of drama and incident today. A massive husky dog suddenly appeared and chased us up the road. Rhys got badly dehydrated in the hot sun. He was on the verge of collapse. We staggered back in 3 hours 10 minutes. I love running in my home patch. I waved at and high-fived so many people I knew. And some I didn't. Very few people turn down a high-five if offered. I felt like Rocky Balboa.

Friday 22 April

Now *that* was a wedding. Alex and Thom had their ceremony in Caerphilly Castle. Seldom have Anna and I partied and laughed so hard. Everyone was just up for it. The castle was crawling with Alex's journalist pals so I was in my element. She is the finest human being I've ever sat next to in a work context. She is one of the most generous, Jesus-like atheists I know. They were special times in the *Press* newsroom. I remember her discreetly pointing out the small ginger lad with the cool haircut from promotions who'd asked her out on a date. Now she's his wife. Funny how life works out.

Anna and I slurped gallons of peach Prosecco and strolled round the castle grounds. Our table was a riot. Between all the laughs and the banter, I was inundated with questions about God. The dancefloor was electric. I put my tie round my head, followed by Thom's dad and every other bloke in there. We gave it loads of air guitar and did a massive conga. Alex put on our song from those infamous newsroom nights out, 'All These Things That I've Done' by The Killers. Anna looked glorious in a tight red dress. I soberly realized at one point that I'm punching well above my weight. There was an awful lot of joy in Caerphilly Castle tonight.

Sunday 24 April

Darren was baptized tonight. He has come a very long way. I remember meeting him during my first week working for St Paul's Church. I had recognized him immediately from the stories I'd written in the *Press*. His broken nose, huge square jaw and eyes that were slightly off centre were unmistakable.

Darren's reputation for drunken violence was legendary. His rap sheet was pages long. He was one of the poster boys of 'feral' teenagers in York. And now he was sitting in the church café area eating Maureen's Battenberg. I knew instinctively that if I went over to talk to him I would become part of his life. That he would need a heavy personal investment. There was a chance, too, that he remembered me as the hack who exposed some of his offences in the paper. That might not have ended well.

It took a while but I did go over. We did bond. I did get too involved. He was an absolute nightmare at times. And yet here we were at his baptism. There always seems to be a wonderful symmetry to the way God works. I see now why he compelled me to sit with Darren that day. In some ways my work with him became redemptive for all those times I crossed the line as a reporter. For all those lives we exposed on the front page. Through journeying with Darren, God helped me see the complexity of one broken life but also the potential for redemption. I don't know how many more times Darren will be arrested, but I do know he has discovered and understands the love of Christ in his life.

For one terrifying moment I thought Darren hadn't grasped the etiquette of full immersion baptism. As the congregation waited for him by the paddling pool, I popped my head in to the choir vestry to walk him out. Darren was butt naked. 'Er, Darren, you do know that you need to wear clothes for this?' I told him. Once the dunking was done I kissed him on the forehead and prayed. I looked around at his church friends and supporters who now work so hard to keep him off the booze and out of prison. It was a beautiful sight. How could I ever doubt God on nights like this?

Wednesday 27 April

Esther and Heidi held each other's hands as they breastfed tonight. It melted me. I could watch them suckle, bubble and burp for hours. When I see a sight as beautiful and delicate as this it helps me believe in God. It is divinely inspired. Surely, two random colliding stars could not have created something so wondrous and profound as a breastfeeding mother?

Thursday 28 April

I'm reading a biography about Hull's favourite son, William Wilberforce. He endured years and years of hopeless rejection and failure in his struggle to end the slave trade. It must have been a strain just to rouse himself every morning and carry on the fight. His friend John Wesley sent him a beautiful letter of encouragement after another anti-slavery bill was defeated. He wrote:

Unless God has raised you up for this very thing, you will be worn out by the opposition of men and devils. But if God be for you, who can be against you? Are all of them together stronger than God? O be not weary of well doing. Go on, in the name of God and in the power of His might.

In all our endeavours to wake the sleeping giant of a church that is Holy Trinity, we must cling to this truth. It's what will rouse us every morning.

Friday 29 April

We were glued to the Royal Wedding coverage all day. I'm full of admiration for the Bishop of London. I don't care how confident you are, how frilly your clerical robes, or how expensive your education, preaching a sermon to two billion people is a tough gig. I'm guessing he wore some extra underpants. Purple ones, probably.

Saturday 30 April

Reading the Bible from start to finish continues to shock and surprise. I read this corker from Deuteronomy 25.11–12 this morning: 'If two men are fighting and the wife of one of them comes to rescue her husband from his assailant, and she reaches out and seizes him by his private parts, you shall cut off her hand. Show her no pity.'

Sunday 1 May

Anna and I have cleared out the loft in preparation for our move to Hull. It was wonderfully cathartic. Waves of nostalgia swept over us as we leafed through my old photos, keepsakes and press cuttings. It painted a picture of the person I used to be. I'm not sure I liked him very much.

Anna found the journal I kept of my inter-railing trip round Europe with Ben in the summer of 1994. It's painful to read now. I was a hormonal, insecure car crash of an 18-year-old. Rarely does my journal touch on the significance of exploring Europe's great cities or the adventurous joy of foreign travel. It's all about which girls looked hot that day, how much beer we'd drunk, and whether I'd managed to avoid a bust-up with the long-suffering Ben. Was I really that shallow?

Monday 2 May

Esther drove us insane this afternoon with her incessant crying. I walked the girls to Mum's to try and make it stop. Grandma was there, thank goodness. Nestling the girls against her ample bosoms stopped their racket almost immediately. She is the baby whisperer.

Thursday 5 May

Rhys and I have passed our marathon fundraising target of £1,000 for Cancer Research. The only downside is that we've got to run the damn thing. I feel like my hamstrings will twang at any moment. Folk have really got on board with it. I've also been made captain of the Cranmer football team for our game against the St John's College students. I'm taking it a bit too seriously.

Friday 6 May

I met up with Neal in Hull today to talk about my role at Holy Trinity. I can tell he is desperate for the cavalry to arrive. We got excited about the potential for growth. He wants me to dream crazy dreams for what this huge building could be used for. There's a gentleness and kindness about Neal that makes me want to cradle him, stroke his thinning hair, and tell him that all will be well. We will be the classic odd couple.

Neal warned me that the bars and clubs surrounding Holy Trinity are wild at weekends with marauding drinkers. And that's just the women. He wondered if I'd want to get involved in the Street Angels project starting up soon in the area. They offer support, water and flip-flops to hammered revellers. I said my calling was more about building relationships inside the pubs rather than outside in a high-vis jacket. He raised his eyebrows at that point. In a good way, I hope. I left Hull with a spring in my step and hope in my heart.

Saturday 7 May

I'm encouraging everyone I know to watch *Of Gods and Men*. It's a true story about the final days of a community of French Trappist monks in Algeria. Muslim extremists are wreaking havoc in the village they serve. The film is basically about whether they flee or stay with the people. One scene affected me in particular. The monks are sitting in silence round the dinner table waiting to be fed. The camera pans round them. They look terrified. The extremists could burst in at any moment. Without saying a word, one of the older brothers puts on a beautiful piece of classical music. He pours each one of them a glass of wine. Slowly their faces become unburdened. It's like the Spirit of God moves among them. They sit and love each other with their expressions. Some smile, some cry. It is an intimate, tender moment. They know God is with them. It truly is a holy communion. Not long after, many of the brothers are kidnapped and murdered. I have goose bumps just writing this. It captures something of the essence of what it means to know and follow Jesus Christ.

Monday 9 May

I can hear Paul telling his teenage daughter off on the phone next door. From what I can make out she has fallen out with her sister over them sharing a room together. It's giving me a glimpse into the future with Esther and Heidi.

We began a two-week teaching block on death and dying today. We went through how to conduct an appropriate funeral visit. Asking how the bereaved families 'feel' seems to be the main question to avoid. We were later given a tour of a local crematorium. Our guide was straight out of a Hammer horror film. He seemed to take a bit too much pleasure in showing us the ovens.

Tuesday 10 May

My mind wandered during a boring bit at college Communion tonight. I reflected on Thom and Alex's wedding in Caerphilly. It gave me a flavour of what I think the Kingdom of God is like. There was nothing secular about that wedding. It was intensely spiritual – bursting with life, fun and generosity. The guests were open and friendly. Our conversations were alive, honest and deep. We ate, drank, laughed and danced. For those few hours we were one. There was love and community among strangers. Yes, the rivers of free Prosecco helped, but what a contrast to the service I went to earlier that morning at a church near the castle. It was dingy, dull and tired. The welcome was cold. There was no sense of joy or holiness. The vicar seemed weary and distant. It felt like he was doing us a favour just being there.

I'm convinced that Jesus – given a choice – would have been on the dance floor with a tie round his head at Thom and Alex's wedding rather than at that service. Only when we grasp this will our churches begin to grow again. I guess my prayer for Holy Trinity is that it will eventually begin to feel a bit like Alex and Thom's wedding. I'm convinced the Kingdom of God is more like a wedding than a traditional church service. The Bible tells me so.

Wednesday 11 May

We toured a local funeral directors today. The only certainty in life is that we'll all end up lying in one. We were given permission to view the deceased body of an elderly Eastern European woman. It's something we'll have to get used to. I found it surreal and unsettling. I tried to imagine what her life was like. What made her laugh? What was her favourite flavour of ice cream? Death is hard to process.

I inevitably thought about my own mortality. I'm guessing the others did too. We stood beside her body praying for her family. We gave thanks for her life. The funeral director was potty. His practical joking is legendary round here. I guess you need a sense of humour to work in a place like that. His favourite gag was to hide in the slide-in fridges and jump out at the young pathologists. I bet they loved him for it after an eight-hour shift.

Bob Dylan's lyrics inspired my prayers in chapel this morning. He is the psalmist for modern times. I read out a line from 'Not Dark Yet' before praying for those suffering from depression, loneliness and bereavement: 'Don't even hear a murmur of a prayer, It's not dark yet, but it's getting there.' I also used words from 'The Ballad of Hollis Brown', 'Chimes of Freedom' and 'I Believe in You'.

Rhys Thomas and I strolled by the river tonight to get mentally ready for Sunday's marathon. He shared the story of how he came to faith. He found God in the shower. What better place to get spiritually clean?

Sunday 15 May

Only I could fall out with someone while running a marathon. Rhys and I had a bust-up 13 miles into the Druridge Bay Marathon. All the energy had drained out of me. Every part of me wanted to quit. Rhys kept going off ahead to make a point that I was denying him a decent time. It tested our pact to stay together no matter what.

The 26 miles included a beach section. The fine sand finished me. Rhys was frustrated but my body had gone. We were desperate to run under 4 hours but it was beyond me. I shouted at him that he should go off on his own because it felt like I was running alone anyway. He refused. We stopped and stared at each other fiercely by a rickety fence. He swore. I swore. We carried on. We ran in furious silence for a mile before laughing about our stupidity. I apologized. He apologized. We carried on. Times became irrelevant and we began to enjoy it.

We'd gathered at Rhys's at 6 a.m. for black coffee and as much pasta as we could eat. We were nervous and tense. Wendy and Liz drove us to the venue and supported us all day with drinks, Midget Gems and words of encouragement. I never want to lay eyes on Druridge Bay again. I don't want to ever hear that name mentioned. Its marathon was physically cruel. The last few miles were utterly hideous. Aunty Lynne kept popping into my head. Her sun-tanned smile. This was for her today.

My bromance with Rhys reached fever pitch in the last mile. I thanked him for his generosity and patience. All those conversations, laughs and prayers during our 5.30 a.m. training runs had come down to this. I felt so close to him. We linked arms and crossed the line together before collapsing on the ground. Twenty-six miles run for Aunty Lynne. £1,200 raised for Cancer Research. A kindred spirit made. A body raging at me never to put it through such appalling trauma ever again.

Thursday 19 May

My clerical clothes arrived today. I stared at the black Matrix-style robe with the 39 buttons, the white, flowing surplice, black shirt and dog collar for a long time before trying them on. It doesn't feel real. It doesn't feel right. No matter which angle I posed at in front of the mirror, I still felt utterly ridiculous. Who am I trying to kid with this? It's not me. Anna tried her best to be supportive but I could see the incredulity in her face. I'm not ready for this. What will people think when I have to wear these clothes in public?

Friday 20 May

Rob and his mate Stagg felted our garage roof today. Stagg is an ex-con who has spent time in a lot of prisons. Apparently he finally turned his life around after looking at the countryside through the bars of his jail cell. It was his epiphany moment. Stagg was fascinated by me becoming a vicar. 'Is there any hope for me?' he asked later. What a privilege to unpack that question with him over a brew and some ginger nuts.

Saturday 21 May

It was our first car boot sale today. We made £2.

Monday 23 May

Today I had a meeting with Tina, one of Cranmer's most experienced pastoral priests. She'd offered to advise me about how I can avoid conflict in a church context. She was blunt and honest enough to be really helpful. Sometimes I need the truth bludgeoned into me. 'Basically, Matt, you need to learn to zip your mouth,' she said. Tina said that some of my verbal outbursts were not appropriate for a priest. 'You are fast, strong and full on, so need to take little steps in order to stop yourself becoming too extreme. You need to practise until they become good habits.' Her advice sounded achievable. Tina thinks my vocabulary is too forceful and direct. She suggested that I learnt to speak more tentatively and increase my quiet periods. My usual words like 'need' and 'must' could be changed to 'ought' and 'should', Tina said.

I felt like Eliza Doolittle in *My Fair Lady* being schooled by Rex Harrison. Tina had me by the emotional short and curlies.

I admitted my distress at putting on the clerical clothes. Tina helped me to see it in a new light. 'Bring Jesus into the conversation,' she said. 'Where is he when you look in the mirror? What is he thinking when you are robed up? Receive his gaze, ask him to speak to you.' I realized in that moment that Jesus would be proud of me. He would look at me like a father looks at his son in their first school play. It was a beautiful thought. I'll carry it with me. I came out of the session full of confidence. I'm determined to be calmer, and gentler with a mouth that zips more frequently.

Friday 27 May

I've received some unbelievable feedback about my assessed sermon. I feel hugely affirmed but also a bit embarrassed. Taking compliments has never been a strong point. Our preaching guru Kate has opened up a whole new world of creativity to me. She refuses to kowtow to the normal preaching conventions. It's why her sermons always feel like an event. Kate will try pretty much anything to communicate the love of God. Sometimes she even preaches from the pulpit. Holy Trinity needs to brace itself. When I leave Cranmer, how Kate does it will be how I strive to do it. With bells on. What a gift this place has been.

Sunday 29 May

If you can't have a family bust-up in church where can you have one? We all went into emotional meltdown today. I felt like I was unravelling. The weight of the impending ordination is a lot to bear. We got off to a bad start. Getting the girls ready for church was the stuff of nightmares. By some miracle we made it to St Paul's but then Anna and I had a row at the back over each other's parenting deficiencies. Mum got involved so I gave her both barrels for interfering. During the sermon I silently fumed. Mum reached out and held my hand. A lot was said in that gesture.

Anna and I had a heart-to-heart over some wine tonight. I expressed how scared I felt about being a vicar. She was brilliant. I sometimes forget that this is her calling too. We are in it together as a family. Anna has to cope with being a vicar's wife, for crying out loud. We laughed at what that could mean for her. I said if she's going to do it properly, she'll need more flowery dresses, a greater willingness to bake and a much larger bottom.

Monday 30 May

I'm so lucky to have Robin Gamble as a mentor. He reassured me that the way I'm feeling is perfectly normal. He understands that I'm an extreme personality. His advice was simple: 'Cleave to Jesus. Cleave to Anna.' Robin said that in ministry there would be thousands of good times and many bad times. 'It's a tough gig,' he said, 'but one full of life at the glory of God. The fact he chooses to use the likes of us to do his work should be a wonderful surprise and a great privilege.' Robin told me that even after 35 years he still gets a buzz going out into the parish in his dog collar as 'God's man'.

Wednesday 1 June

Dad visited me in Durham today. It was spiritually significant. At a college barbecue he opened up to Bill about Jesus. After a long, intense conversation, Bill looked him in the eyes and said: 'You need to forgive yourself, John.' Dad wept.

Sunday 5 June

Not only am I not producing enough sperm to be useful, now the little I do have is coming out too flipping quickly. I've developed a bit of an issue with premature ejaculation. I'm hoping it's just a phase. Anna tried so hard not to look disappointed this afternoon. She stroked my back like I was really ill or something.

She described me as the 'love of her life'. It was amazing to hear those words. It made me feel warm and wonderful inside.

Monday 6 June

Sister Cecilia says that when we are on the verge of doing big things for God, we can come under spiritual attack. She may be right. Weird things keep happening to me at night. I suffered a fairly dark, terrifying experience in my college room in the early hours today. I woke to discover some sort of faceless black form in the middle of the room. It hovered for a while. Then I heard a piercing scream. It was like something from *Harry Potter*. I was half asleep but don't think I imagined it. I resisted the temptation to climb in with Paul next door for a reassuring man spoon. Instead, I laid in fear for a while before finally dropping off. At the weekend I kept dreaming that the babies were being snatched from us. I now hold my cross and pray for Christ's protection and peace before I go to sleep.

Paul treated me to a fish foot spa this morning. They are special little tiddlers that nibble at your feet to clear away the dead skin and impurities. They went straight for my big toe. It was a feeding frenzy! We belly-laughed at the strangely comforting tickling sensation. The place was run by two salt-of-the-earth Geordie lasses. I wondered if the fish had swum in off the back of a lorry. Once the fish were full of my toe fungus, one of the girls said (with a straight face): 'If you'd now like to make your way to the dedicated drying area, please.' It consisted of two soggy hand towels on the floor in the corner of the room. I love that.

Every moment with Paul is precious now. Our lives will never be the same again once we're revs. We're realistic enough to know that our time and weekends will be gobbled up. I treated Paul to a scone afterwards. He ordered extra cream. Greedy.

The St John's College students stuffed us 11–2 in the big footy match this afternoon. It was only 4–2 at half time. Loads of staff and ordinands came to support us. Joel Wood was our man of the match. He played with the intensity and fire of the prophet Elijah. I'd handed out a shirt to each of our players beforehand in the changing rooms like a proper manager. They lapped it up. I can't remember actually touching the ball but I shouted and encouraged the team a lot.

I had a significant spiritual encounter with two post-graduate students in Osbournes tonight. Steve and Alex are inquisitive guys. We'd been building to this all term. They opened up for the first time about their life and faith. Steve asked me to share my favourite Gospel story. I chose the one from John 6. It's where many of Jesus' disciples have deserted him. He turns to Peter and says: 'You do not want to leave too, do you?' Peter replies: 'Lord, to whom shall we go? You have the words of eternal life.' I encouraged the lads that they are brilliant, learned young men. They're restless seekers of truth. They hoover up books, join in debates, and dissect the latest fashionable philosophies. But once you experience Jesus for real, I said, there's nowhere else to look. He is it. I explained that I had a Peter moment. I experienced his truth and love in my life. 'It changed everything,' I said. 'And now here we are.' It was a holy moment. The lads quietly sipped their beer. Nothing more needed to be said.

Tuesday 7 June

I had my final tutorial with Stuart. We've had quite a journey together. He taught me a lot. He is a fine priest with a superb haircut. Stuart presented me with a lovely book of healing and wholeness prayers. Inside he wrote: 'As you prepare to leave college and be ordained as a deacon, this little book is a reminder of God's gift of healing and wholeness to you. I pray that you would be a channel of his healing and wholeness in a hurting and broken world.'

I received my lowest mark of the year today for the systematics structured conversation. The marker accused me of waffling and a 'pick and mix' approach to the atonement. Fair enough. It means that overall I was 1.5 per cent off a distinction. I'm happy with that. I've worked hard. Learning all this theology has been a hard-fought gift. My faith has been stretched. It has evolved, matured even. I'm less spiritually naïve but just as hope-filled. I've got a few more questions for God when I see him. Two years of intense theological training has boiled down to this: the Christian faith really is all a beautiful mystery. But the answer is still Jesus. Thank God for that.

Wednesday 8 June

Our final college quiet day on Holy Island was a melancholy time. I found a nice spot and wrote cards to all the Cranmer staff who have particularly impacted me. The list included tutors, teachers, cleaners and cooks. It was therapeutic to recall memories and experiences I'd forgotten in the mania of college and family life. I drew a cartoon for my conflict guru, Tina. It depicted Archbishop Sentamu tying a gag over my mouth.

Inevitably I walked to the rock where I proposed to Anna. It was spoiled by an old couple scoffing their sandwiches nearby. Every time I settled into a nice vibe their two scruffy dogs barked at me. I walked away. The day finished with a poignant service in St Mary's Church. We were invited to dip our fingers into the font and make the sign of the cross on the forehead of someone who had prayed for us at Cranmer. It was a bit awkward at first but turned into something very special. Aidan made a beeline for my head with his finger. I crossed Jason, Rob and Stuart among others but I was spoilt for choice. Many of this group have prayed for me. I was grateful for all of them.

I've received a delightful card from my student neighbour on B Floor, Zach. He wrote: 'You've been an incredible mate to me. I have to say it has made a huge difference to my time here to have you down the corridor. I hope that wherever you go in the future you will continue to bring life, good humour and copious amounts of idiocy.' How lovely. It shows there's real power in a half-decent Stevie Wonder impression.

Thursday 9 June

Christ came to me in a really special way at the leavers' service tonight. I could 'feel' how proud he is of me for following his call. I wasn't conscious of anyone else in the room. Just me and him. I've been making jokes at my own expense since the robes arrived. It has been my way of running from the seriousness and responsibility of my calling. Christ turned that on its head tonight. I see myself differently now. I cried quiet tears during the service. Jesus is proud of me. I know that now. Those of us leaving Cranmer were invited forward for prayer. We were given a lighted candle as a symbol of us being sent out.

Earlier, David treated those of us on the common room committee to a final lunch. The place was quite swish so we were conservative with our orders. Except Jason. He was shameless. Starters, extra wine, a dessert with an unpronounceable name. Money was no object. I imagine the colour drained from David's face when he got the bill.

Friday 10 June

This is it. My last day at Cranmer. There's nothing more they can teach me now. I've made it without walking out or being chucked out. I learned far more than theology here. I've grown to love the place and the people with a special passion. There was a lovely moment after Morning Prayer when all the stayers formed a guard of honour and clapped out the leavers. We then returned the compliment. We gave a special cheer to our warden, David. He looked well chuffed. David is the eccentric uncle I always wanted. I'd go over hot coals for him.

It was also Morning Glory's final prayer meeting. Sanjay, Rob, Jason and Aidan. I'd never have chosen them as close friends but now I wouldn't be without them. Even Aidan. They are my brothers. We each said what the group had meant to us and shared our favourite memory. My biggest achievement was that I managed to stay in the group. There were times when I wanted to be anywhere else on a Thursday morning. The lads persevered with me. So many of our prayers were answered. As the two leavers, Sanjay and I knelt down while the other lads laid hands on us and prayed. Then we had one last wrestle. We've agreed to keep meeting up for a Morning Glory retreat twice a year. We'll need it.

My time at Cranmer ended appropriately – with a party. It's what Jesus would have wanted. There was a live band, hog roast and gallons of Pimms with those annoying bits of mint in it. I borrowed Jason's ludicrously expensive tailored jacket to go with my only decent shirt. He drunkenly said I could have it as a leaving gift. He'll regret that in the morning. I collared our college principal David to draw from his massive intellect one last time. 'Any final words of wisdom?' I asked. 'Be yourself!' he replied. He surely can't mean that?!

It all got very emotional as the night wore on. There was way too much hugging. I've now fled the slurred farewells in an effort to find some stirring words to sum up my time here. I can't muster any. The last word should be to God. Thank you for my time at Cranmer. You knew what you were doing. I need to lie down. Quickly.

Saturday 11 June

I received a classic text from Aidan this morning. He is a drama queen, king and prince all rolled into one. I dread to think what slurred drivel came out of my mouth in our conversations at the party last night to warrant such a message. It says: 'Goodbye, Matt. I have never and will never stop loving you. Our "problems" are a figment of your imagination and I have forgiven anything you think you've done wrong to me (although I'm still not clear what they may be). I'm sorry for the many times I've inadvertently p****d you off!' Only at theological college could I have forged a close bond with a guy like Aidan. We are so different. I'm relieved we got through it without physical harm coming to either one of us. I'm a better person for knowing him.

Driving out of Durham I'd planned to pray some big, dramatic prayers, like a spiritual cowboy riding off into the sunset for his next adventure. I had a lot to thank God for – not least that he put incredible people across my path these last two years. I'll always cherish them. To be honest, though, I got distracted trying to prise out those annoying bits of mint from my teeth. They weren't shifting. I was in York before I knew it and the moment had gone.

Three glorious smiles were waiting to greet me at home. My girls were all packed and ready for a week's holiday to Bamburgh with Rob and Sarah, Anna's parents and the kids. The thought of all of us being cooped up in a cottage hasn't made my heart sing. Paul and Sue have been off with me lately. More than usual. It's time for us to get on. This could be the holiday to make it right once and for all. I'm looking forward to unveiling the new Matt. He's more tolerant, patient, respectful, low-maintenance and humble. Conflict is the way of the old Matt. We can do a week of peace and harmony, surely?

Sunday 12 June

Tension is mounting. My tongue is bloodied and blistered from all the biting. Paul and Sue are clearly very unhappy with me. Their displeasure and disapproval leak out at every opportunity. Something is going to blow. It feels like they have stored up a year's worth of frustration at me being away from Anna and the girls at college. Maybe they're also upset at the fact that I'm taking them away to live in Hull. I understand their feelings. Up to a point. I can't be an easy person to have your precious daughter married to. I just wish they'd have it out with me properly. Instead, there's an awful simmering tension in the cottage. I keep finding places to hide. If my early nights get any earlier I'll be hitting the sack at lunchtime. The hardest place to be a Christian – let alone a reverend – is with your family. Fact.

Tuesday 14 June

This holiday can't end soon enough. Paul's criticisms of me have reached a new level of creativity and comedy. I was giving the girls a drink of water, so he quipped: 'Don't give them water – you'll drown them!' I know that I've been really difficult in the past. I've said and done things I shouldn't have in their company. But St Cuthbert would have lost his temper and sworn by now. I can sense they are as frustrated with me as I am with them. We are united by our love for Anna and the girls, but not a lot else right now. I just wish this tension would lift. It's a shame because Bamburgh is a stunning place with a fantastic beach. Anna is permanently on edge. She's self-medicating with Pinot Grigio.

Thursday 16 June

This was the day when the gloves came off. When things were said that we always wanted to say but never dared. Bamburghgate was born today. I'd done pretty well keeping out of Paul and Sue's way up to this point. The frostiness had reached arctic levels by late afternoon. I went out for a walk. When I got back I could hear Anna and Sue shouting at each other. It was loud. Instinctively, I knew this was the time to have it out once and for all. I ran into the room and waded in. I felt like the 'other' woman storming onto the *Jerry Springer* set for a showdown. Sue's face was red with fury. She accused me of ruining the holiday. 'I could say exactly the same thing!' I snapped back. She lost it. I think I was close to being hit at that point.

We sat down. With a surprisingly calm head, I asked them to give it to me straight. What were their issues? 'List them,' I demanded. Paul said it would take hours. At my insistence, he began to list a catalogue of stuff. In no particular order: I'm the most selfish person he's ever met; I fall out with *everyone*; I only ever talk about myself; they bend over backwards to make it work with me. It went on. Paul had really given this some thought. For the most part, I took his litany of criticisms without arguing back. Some of what he said was true and fair. Some of it wasn't. But it was important that Paul vented his spleen. I'm glad he did. His resentment had clearly been years in the making.

My mouth didn't stay completely shut, mind you. I told Sue at one point that 'if I never see you again it will be too soon'. It was an awful thing to say. I regretted saying it and immediately apologized. I know I was never their favourite choice to be Anna's husband but I hadn't realized their dislike ran so deep. I asked Paul if he had any flaws that needed working on. His reply was pithy to say the least: 'No. I can't think of any.' I apologized for some of the things on Paul's list. There was nothing left to say. That's where we left it. We are leaving in the morning. Anna sobbed herself to sleep.

Friday 17 June

Before we left, I had another round of talks with Sue. I hoped we could make progress. We didn't. I asked her how she thought we could move on as a family. 'We'll just have to put up with you and get on with it,' she replied. 'How about a family mediator?' I suggested. She left the room at that point. Do Paul and Sue know that Anna and I are quite happily married?

Driving away from that oppressive atmosphere was such a relief. Anna cried all the way home. She's stuck right in the middle. I'm really trying to understand how we got to this point. Their issues with me probably go way back to when Paul was my youth leader at church. I was a nightmare at that age. The seeds of Paul's discontent were probably sown on those Friday nights when he would have to kick me out of the youth club every week. Apparently, he actually said to Derek the vicar after one particularly unfortunate incident involving a pool cue and a leader's front tooth: 'I pity who ever marries that boy!' It must have felt like a *very* long walk up that church aisle with Anna on our wedding day.

Saturday 18 June

Anna is distraught. I suggested we go to see her parents tomorrow for another round of talks. If we don't deal with this now, it could be years before we are reconciled. We're all stubborn people.

I don't want this situation to fester or a cancer of bitter resentment will grow and spread. Everything is out in the open now. We've got to move on for the sake of Anna and the babies. I'm trying hard to see things from their perspective. I know I'm far from easy.

Mum came round with a Rastafarian wig on to cheer me up. We danced and sang 'No Woman, No Cry' in the worst Caribbean accent ever.

Sunday 19 June

Diplomatic relations have been restored with Paul and Sue. Peace has prevailed. Love has won the day. Before going round, Anna and I prayed hard for the right words, receptive hearts and a way forward. From the moment we walked through the door the atmosphere was positive. Of course the elephant was allowed to sit in their lounge for ages before anyone mentioned it. We are English after all. We were all being so polite and careful. Eventually I blurted out: 'Well, you'll all be pleased to know that I've booked us into the cottage again next year.' It thawed the room. I apologized for my part in Bamburghgate. I meant it too.

Searching for some words and answers in the shower that morning, an epiphany moment came. I focused on putting myself in their shoes. It was an uncomfortable place to stand. A clear picture emerged. I saw that Paul and Sue have carried a lot for us these past few months. Too much. They have sacrificed so much for us. For me. They pretty much took on my role supporting Anna and the babies mid-week while I was at Cranmer. My forced absence did not make their heart grow fonder. Neither did my somewhat *laissez-faire* approach to childcare and house-husbandry when I returned home at weekends. And now I'll be riding off into the sunset with their beloved daughter and grandchildren.

Paul and Sue are good people. As parents and grandparents they are utterly reliable, patient, loving and solid. I need to start learning from them, not resenting them. Starting today. Yes, Paul and Sue could have handled Bamburgh differently. They could have said something. Cleared the air. But that's not their way. Stepping out of the shower and back into my own shoes, I knew what I needed to do. Apologize. Unreservedly and without condition. To name what I'd done, not done and when I'd expected them to do too much. And that's what I did. I thanked them too. I found myself really loving them as these conciliatory words came out of my mouth. It was a holy moment. A lovely peace descended. I instinctively know that things will be better between us now. More guarded perhaps, but better.

Anna's face unfurrowed for the first time in weeks. Paul and Sue were apologetic in their own way. Sue admitted that she came close to clocking me somewhere painful. We joked about me trying to explain a big shiner at my pre-ordination meeting with Archbishop Sentamu tomorrow. 'I've had some issues with my mother-in-law, Archbishop!' It was nice to laugh with them again. Reconciliation is awesome. Being a Christian really does work in practice. Even with your in-laws.

Monday 20 June

I dared myself to be brutally honest with Archbishop Sentamu at our crunch meeting this morning. Technically, he could still have called my ordination off. This was the meeting when he finally decides if I'm priest material or not. I suppose it's like when the X-Factor contestants go to the judges' houses to discover if they are being put through to the live final. Except I was in a palace and my judge is way tougher than Simon Cowell. So when Sentamu asked how I was, I swallowed hard and went for it. 'I've been having a nightmare, Archbishop!' I gave him the edited highlights of Bamburghgate. Sentamu broke out into one of his glorious gap-toothed smiles. 'That's why they're called the outlaws!' he said. What a legend.

The meeting was a joy after that. He asked what I'd got out of the whole Cranmer experience. I said the academic study was enriching but it was the community life that I'd learnt the most from. We got onto some of my doctrinal struggles and the importance of getting the balance right between theological study and putting it into practice. He reminded me that it wasn't just

Anna's job to bring up the twins. Before I went, he looked me straight in the eye and said, 'Never forget, Matt, that Jesus is your friend.' My body became covered in goose bumps at the truth of his words. With that, the Archbishop said he accepted me for ordination. We move to Hull tomorrow.

Tuesday 21 June

We are now residents of Kingston-upon-Hull. The big move wasn't as horrible as we predicted. Saying goodbye to our house in Glebe Avenue was hard. It's home. The next time we live there will probably be when I'm drawing a pension. Our new neighbours seem friendly. We live about 100 metres from the banks of the Humber. There's a lovely walkway and cycle path beside it. I sound like an estate agent. I'm trying to be positive but it's hard. We're hurting and a bit scared.

I've received my official letter of confirmation from Archbishop Sentamu. He wrote: 'You have been at Cranmer for two years during which the training, formation and academic study have stretched you. I think that this has been positive in terms of your development, and I hope that activism will not subsume all you have been learning while at Cranmer ... As a pioneer minister you have always got to be prepared to go where others feel God is calling you to go. Like Abraham, you must always have a faith ready for adventure, not always knowing where you are going, but glad to go wherever God is calling you to serve.'

My impending ordination is doing funny things to my friends. Pete sent me a text that was very unlike him. He wrote: 'OK, sounds weird this, buddy, but I've had this massive strong urge to pray for you all against spiritual attacks and stuff so, erm, stay strong!' I'm surrounded by incredible blokes. Holy Trinity's churchwarden, Tim Wilson, popped in to see us. I liked him instantly. His eyes sparkled with wit and mischief. We'll get on.

Tonight we washed a Chinese down with a bottle of champagne to celebrate our move. Classy. Anna looks terrified.

Wednesday 22 June

Mum is over to stay so we can get the house sorted. She came back despondent after visiting Holy Trinity. One of the church welcomers told her all about the building's historical treasures. When she asked about worship he was very keen to tell her that he wasn't part of that. She didn't say it, but I can tell Mum is wondering why I've agreed to serve at such a difficult church. I need her to believe in me that I can do this.

My new boss Neal came round with a card and a bottle of red wine. The more I see him, the more I like him. His eyes looked weary. I get the impression he's working himself too hard. My first job will be to give him a lift. Blind passion and enthusiasm can be infectious. Neal was feeling bruised after a heated debate with the church council last night over whether to introduce candles to Holy Trinity. Neal is adamant that people should be able to light one in the prayer chapel. Apparently some of the church stalwarts are worried that lighting candles is too Catholic. So, Holy Trinity's pews are virtually empty on Sundays, there's little or no community engagement, and it's close to financial ruin. The church council is debating the rights and wrongs of candles. It's going to be a long road.

Thursday 23 June

I spent a much-needed retreat day at the Bede Centre with Sister Cecilia. Being with her always draws me closer to God. I leave her knowing God just a little bit better than when I first arrived. Cecilia helps to explain and 'normalize' my dark nights of the soul. She took particular interest in my God encounter during the leavers' retreat weekend. She thinks it gave me 'the graces' to handle the aftermath of Bamburghgate. I was encouraged to read one of her pamphlets today called *Crisis of Faith: Danger or Opportunity?* It was so relevant to my recent experiences. Cecilia writes: 'to use the terminology of the mystics we are touching moments of the "Prayer of the Quiet" when God enters into our lives tangibly and mysteriously. We understand very little that we can put into words, yet we are changed and "held" by that experience.' Cecilia talks about 'hollowing out' to allow space for the divine encounter: 'we are being hollowed out for God in two ways: firstly we are being enabled to let go of so many props and supports that have in the past symbolized God for us. Instead, we are being invited to stand in the stark emptiness of God's own presence and to allow God to teach us the way.' Cecilia says that during this process we may act in very ungodly ways. Our libidos may increase, we may drink more (so that explains it!). She continues: 'It is as if we are being hollowed out but at first cannot understand how to cope – or how to satisfy the yearning … what I believe is happening is that we are being given a second chance to revisit parts of our deepest selves that once we could not handle or integrate.'

I marvel at Cecilia's earthiness. She has a gift of rooting the experiences, trials and joys of our spiritual lives into our everyday lives. This stuff makes sense to me. My heart can grasp it. I drove back to Hull feeling refreshed and reassured. And more than a little hollowed out.

Friday 24 June

I ran 5 miles round the streets of East Hull this morning. It's interesting that the poorer an area is, the more bookies and moneylenders there are. Anna will be pleased there's a Home Bargains nearby. I was so proud of her today. I accompanied her to the twins' club at our local community centre. She was in mummy heaven. She told me to leave after five minutes. That's always a good sign. Anna has finally found a group of women who have been through the same thing as her. She loved it. What a relief.

Sunday 26 June

In preparation for the big day, I'm reading R. S. Thomas's collection of autobiographical poems, *The Echoes Return Slow*. He was a curmudgeonly, miserable old priest by all accounts, but boy could he write. I could have chosen something cheerier, but his stuff speaks to my deepest places. In one stanza, he brutally articulates the harsh reality of doing a pastoral visit in a tough place. And yet he's still aware of that faint hint of something more profound going on. The small shaft of hope that the encounter in 'the thickening shadows of their kitchens' could have real spiritual value.

Ministry at Holy Trinity will be hard. Gruelling, even. I know that. I'm ready for it. There will be times, I'm sure, to wrap myself in 'the heavier clothes of my calling'. But I'm determined to do all I can to find opportunities to speak of the light and love that comes from knowing Jesus Christ. It's what I'm here to do. It's what I'm called to do.

Wednesday 29 June

Anna had a meltdown today. The full realization that she has moved away hit her hard. She's missing our home, her mum and all the support networks we have in York. This is part of the grieving process of moving away, I guess. Anna said she feels vulnerable and scared. She's not the only one. I made her laugh before we turned in. It felt therapeutic for both of us. I've indulged myself by ordering Sky TV. Jeff Stelling could be my only friend for a while.

Thursday 30 June

I'm at the ordination retreat feeling weird but strangely at peace. I will be turned into a reverend in three days. A clerk in holy orders. I was so glad that Lee dropped me off at the Minster for our run through of the ordination service. We had one of those lovely, intimate friendship moments. He knows how big this is. His best friend is becoming a vicar. That can't be easy to get your head round. Lee brought two of his freshly made pork pies. We ate them noisily on the Minster steps. Heavenly. I bet God was laughing at the sight of us.

We tried to make sense of what I was about to do. We couldn't. With a few final words of encouragement and a fist pump, Lee disappeared into a sea of Japanese tourists. Before I knew it I was standing in a black robe being briefed by the canon responsible for organizing Sunday's service. He immediately put us at ease, which was good because we were all terrified. As he walked us through the different elements of the two-hour service, the enormity of what I was embarking upon hit me afresh. There's a moment during the ceremony when they call out your individual name and title parish. That's the cue to turn to face the congregation. What's still unclear is how our face is supposed to look at that crucial point. I didn't dare ask. Do we smile? Wink? Nod? Wave? Give the thumbs up? I'm too conscious of it now. It's all I could think about.

Later we went on to Bishopthorpe Palace for further briefings. I met Irene Wilson for the first time. We'll be fellow curates together at Holy Trinity. She's wonderful. So refreshingly grounded, good-humoured and up for it. Irene admitted to being apprehensive that I would be some high-flying academic type. I quickly put her straight on that one.

Each of us stood in front of Archbishop Sentamu in his chapel and made our legal declarations. These words actually came out of my mouth: 'I, Matthew Ross Woodcock, do so affirm and accordingly declare my belief in the faith which is revealed in the Holy Scriptures and set forth in the catholic creeds and to which the historic formularies of the Church of England bear witness.'

I felt like I was in a period drama. The diocesan registrar, resplendent in a legal wig and black gown, presented each of us with our papers in the form of a scroll tied with a red ribbon.

A lovely priest is leading our retreat. It's in Hull, as it happens. She's calm, gentle and holy. Just what I need. It's squeaky bum time!

Saturday 2 July

After some lovely sessions peppered with poems and times of reflection, Paul Bromley and I got a bus into town. I wanted to show him our new house and Holy Trinity. He'd calm anyone's nerves. It's strange just going about my business. Life won't ever be the same again after tomorrow. We tried to relax over a few wines in the bar tonight. I was probably too loud. By noon tomorrow I will be forever known as the Reverend Matt Woodcock. I won't be getting a lot of sleep.

Sunday 3 July

I woke up a Mr. I've come to bed a Rev. It's both an incredible privilege and a terrifying reality. It was tense this morning. We all dealt with it in our own way. I called Anna, Mum and Robin for a few final words of encouragement. There were cheers in the breakfast room as each of us came down in our clerical shirts and dog collars. It was like getting ready for the FA Cup Final.

I got to the Minster early to process what was about to happen and practise the choreography. I sat on a stone step out of sight, brooding for one more time about what I was about to do.

We made silly small talk, readjusted our robes, stretched and practised our kneeling technique. Then it all just happened. A scrum of important clergy in an assortment of colours suddenly converged on us. We filed in behind Archbishop Sentamu and processed into the nave to the sound of a deafeningly grand organ piece. It felt like a coronation. I walked next to Irene trying not to tremble or trip over my cassock. Then I became conscious of what facial expression to adopt as I filed past the people. I went for a half-smile in the end but then worried it looked like a self-satisfied smirk. As we marched to the back of the nave my heart soared. I caught sight of some of the Post Office footy lads who'd come to support me. Wellsy and Kaiser looked magnificent in their suits and hair gel. They gave me huge cheesy grins and looked so proud. I swallowed down the tears. Then I spotted the gang – Mum, Grandma, Amy, Dad, Lee, Ian, Ben and Anna.

The service began and we were called out and presented to the Archbishop and archdeacons. We turned to face the people. I made sure I smiled. I was intensely moved as I kneeled before Sentamu at the crunch moment. He laid his hands on my head and said: 'Send down the Holy Spirit on your servant Matthew for the office and work of a deacon in your Church.' Then he anointed my head with oil. In that holy moment I was ordained. I became a reverend.

The rest of the day is a blur. I know there were thousands of snaps taken on the Minster steps. I spent the next six hours in the Fox beer garden saying thank you to everyone in my dog collar. Everyone wanted a pic with the new rev in town. I barely got chance to hold Anna and the girls. What a day. A few years ago I promised God I'd push every door he told me to. It's led me to this. I am the Reverend Matt Woodcock. Lord help us all.

Monday 4 July

I spent the day adjusting to my new title. I'm overwhelmed with people's cards, gifts and supportive Facebook messages. Jason and Ruth bought me a lovely watch. Jason said it was high time I replaced my beloved Casio for a 'proper grown-up's watch'. His card moved me to tears. It sums up so many of my hopes, prayers and fears. He wrote:

It has been a privilege to get to know you and pray with you over these last two years. You are an amazing guy and I'm very excited to see what God is going to do through and with you. Here comes the sermon: Never forget that you are first and foremost a dad and husband. You can do nothing on your own, it is the Spirit who gives you power. Think of others first, don't reply in anger. People genuinely love you and want to be with you, don't be selfish with your time. You are one of the most passionate, genuine prayers I have ever met. Look for what you can learn from people who don't experience God the way you do. Don't ever lose your ability to connect with real people who are lost and hurting – you are great at it. Never forget me. I love you, buddy. Jason.

He's definite bishop material.

It's my first official day as a reverend at Holy Trinity tomorrow. I'll start the day walking the parish with my dog collar on. I'm ready.

Acknowledgements

A large cast of brilliant people – too many to mention – helped and encouraged me to write this book. Anna is chief among them. I don't have the superlatives to sum up all that you've done for and mean to me. Much love always.

And the rest:
Mum, Dad and Amy
Grandma
Uncle Ally, Jo, Beck and Loz.
Uncle Mike, Deb, Ben, Hannah and Rose
Honor, Joely, Phoebe and Keith
My in-laws, Paul and Sue. Fancy Bamburgh next year?
Sarah, Thomas, Elsie and Rob
Matty, Laura and Georgia
Lee and Dave
Jonny 'the Wolf' and Anne. Ben and Ruth (satisfied?!). Ollie. Tan. Woz, Deano... The Growlers
Andy and Tom for that initial kick up the backside
Terry, Paul and Dan
To my honest feedbackers, Andy B, Pete Hale, Dr Kate, Dan Broom
The Morning Glory boys for their care, prayer, and belly laughs
Thomas and all at CHP and Hymns Ancient and Modern
Arun and those hills of Meribah

The sensational people of St Paul's Church, Holgate, and Holy Trinity Church, Hull

Robin and Mo Gamble. Bob and Heather Mapplebeck. Derek Wooldridge. John Young. John Lee

My Holy Trinity friends and colleagues, particularly Revs Neal and Irene for their love and limitless patience

The Alden family for letting me park. Professor Howell A. Lloyd and the University of Hull for use of the library

Carole Ashton for our Horseshoe sessions

Former *York Press* comrades, particularly Alex, Mike, Hitcho, Rich and Gav

The Bishopthorpe Palace team

The @kingcityrevs boys, Ben and Jerome

Matt Commerford for our conversations about truth and stationery

Friends, workers and quaffers in Hull's glorious Old Town (the loveliest part of the most underrated city in Europe), particularly: the early-shift staff at Nero's and Costa for the cheerfulness that came with the Americanos; the Blue Bell Friday gang and Lee and Charlotte at the Minerva

My spiritual guide and inspiration, Sister Cecilia Goodman at The Bede Centre

The Community of the Holy Cross

The cow-field on the outskirts of Criccieth

I remain in awe of Cranmer Hall (it may not have come across at times). The standard of teaching was immense but I learnt so much more than theology there. It's a place to truly get to grips with the essence of Christian community. I will always be indebted to the incredible Cranmer leaders and team.

To all those who helped us bring Esther and Heidi into the world: The IVF nurses and doctors at Leeds General Infirmary. Graeme Urwin. The maternity ward staff at York Hospital. The countless prayers, comforters, financial supporters and never-give-up-hopers. St John of Dringhouses. And Our Father.

Special thanks to Noel, Liam, Bonehead, Tony and Guigsy for making *Definitely Maybe.*

I fully appreciate that some of the people featured in this book may have seen things differently. I have tried hard to disguise the potentially embarrassed, change names and seek permissions where necessary.

This book is written in memory of four special people who really showed me how to live and love – Granddad, Aunty Lynne, Ozzy Winfield and Susie Meakin-Clark.

Nero's, Queen Victoria Square, Hull
July 2016